52 PREPPER
PROJECTS

52 PREPPER PROJECTS

A Project a Week to Help You Prepare for the
Unpredictable

David Nash

Introduction by James Talmage "Dr. Prepper" Stevens

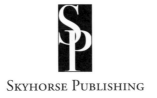

Skyhorse Publishing

Skyhorse Publishing books may be purchased in bulk at special discounts for sales promotion, corporate gifts, fund-raising, or educational purposes. Special editions can also be created to specifications. For details, contact the Special Sales Department, Skyhorse Publishing, 307 West 36th Street, 11th Floor, New York, NY 10018 or info@skyhorsepublishing.com.

Skyhorse® and Skyhorse Publishing® are registered trademarks of Skyhorse Publishing, Inc.®, a Delaware corporation.

www.skyhorsepublishing.com

10 9 8 7

Library of Congress Cataloging-in-Publication Data is available on file.

ISBN: 978-1-61608-849-1

Printed in China

Table of Contents

To my long-suffering wife who let me run a steam engine on her kitchen stove and ruin several of her good pots to melt wax and cook "experiments." She doesn't understand everything I do, but she supports me anyway.

Introduction

I had interviewed David Nash early in January 2013 on one of my Thursday Noon talk shows, and he mentioned he was writing a book organized around weekly prepper-oriented task(s). As I asked more quetsions, it seemed like a great idea and a reasonable method to become prepared without killing your family budget. I urged him to get on the air on the Preparedness Radio Network and share his ideas with our listening audience. He thought about it for a while, then contacted me and agreed to become one of the show's hosts. The rest is truly Internet radio history!

David and I share many of the same points of view on personal and family preparedness. We both believe that getting out and working toward our goals is the only way to prepare for times of hardship. We both realize that just thinking about a project doesn't get it done—but getting started and working toward your goals does.

We also both believe that to prepare for future disasters we need to consider the present knowledge base and utilize the massive amount of information available today—and realize that many of the common past-era or "historical" skills of past generations have a place in modern preparedness planning.

David's book introduces some of those historical skills while also incorporating new ideas gleaned from modern technology. Together they provide a working knowledge that can be developed into several valuable hybrid skills.

The information that became the nucleus of my best-selling book *Making the Best of Basics: Family Preparedness Handbook* came from the generational wisdom of my mother, who passed it on from her mother down through several family generations. David, his native curiosity coupled with his willingness to explore new concepts, also learned the value of being prepared from his mother. Perhaps that's why we both believe that common-sense solutions, applied ingenuity, and a highly developed work ethic are the cornerstones for establishing the foundation for the most important aspects of survival.

I really don't like the term "expert"—I never use it to describe myself. There are too many self-proclaimed "experts" offering advice on preparedness without actually doing what they tell others to do. The only reason I'm writing the foreword to his book is because I perceived that David was not a self-promoting prepper but a truly sincere person willing to develop the best way to get the job done. He is constantly studying, practicing, and developing new (at least to him) skills, talents, and abilities from old concepts with new ideas. What he does is share those experiences with all of us.

When you read this book, those experiences come through and you know he isn't telling you what he read on a random website but, rather, what he has accomplished with his hands.

I have been involved in personal preparedness for a long time——from my first Boy Scout camping trip at the tender age of twelve until now (I am in my mid seventies). I have learned, taught, written about, and practiced disaster preparedness longer than I like to think or remember! My own book, *Making the Best of Basics*, is in its 14th edition and has sold more than 800,000 copies, so I feel I can confidently express what it takes to be an effective prepper. At this point I know what works and what is fluff.

With that said, I think that *52 Prepper Projects,* with all the projects in it and the concepts behind them, is worthy of study and merits a place on any prepper's bookshelf.

James Talmage Stevens / a.k.a "Doctor Prepper"

How to Use This Book

This book is an attempt to organize some of my favorite projects. The idea is that if you are new to "prepping" and/or DIY, it is easy to get overwhelmed and give up without ever doing much more than reading a book or buying a bucket or two of food.

Everybody has limited resources; even the federal government has limitations on how much it can spend on disaster preparedness. So this book will not be about buying a closet full of stuff. It is about how to get the most benefit from the least amount of resources.

The projects in this book are designed to fit in a middle-income family's budget (because that is *my* budget). We did not give up cable or make any extreme lifestyle changes to afford to do these projects, but we did make some sacrifices.

I started with a small amount of hand tools and very little skill. But many of these projects leverage the skills, tools, and devices created previously to allow you to do things in six months that you would never attempt today.

Included along with the weekly projects is an incremental shopping list. I could not afford to go buy everything I needed to feed, clothe, and protect my family in one big shopping spree. But when I just threw a couple random "prepper" items in the shopping cart every trip I both blew up my budget and failed to have a means to track what I was buying and what I still needed to buy. This shopping list allows you to buy a few things each week. It does not noticeably add to your family budget, but after six months you will have a very respectable disaster supply closet.

The shopping list should be worked on simultaneously with the projects in this book. That way as you build skills you are also building a substantial basic disaster kit.

If you follow my blog then you know I follow a tiered concept. I make sure that I balance my preparedness acquisitions so that I have a well-rounded approach to preparedness. This incremental plan does that as well.

The last section is the meat of the book; it contains all the projects. It is designed for you to complete them in order, but most people will probably skip around. All I ask is that you realize that while this is a blueprint that I followed, you are building your own house, so make it work for you. If a project does not fit your lifestyle don't do it, but spend some time thinking about why the project was included and if you need to find a workable replacement for your lifestyle. Not everyone wants to raise small livestock, but everyone needs a protein source.

Incremental Disaster Shopping List

Buying a premade 72-hour kit can be expensive and making one can be intimidating. This weekly shopping list will allow you to put aside a decent emergency preparation kit in about five months by doing a little every seven days. The long-term goal is to be as easy on you and your wallet as possible while helping you create a workable kit.

Once you have a cushion, you'll find that you've managed to prepare yourself and your family for the little things in life that can throw you off track. As you continue, you'll be adding to that piece of mind, and you'll also find less and less situations you're unprepared for. Remember, this kit should be made in addition to, and over and above, what you already have, so even if you have a can opener, when you see it on the list, buy another and put it away with your supplies.

Week 1 Shopping List

To Buy:

- ❏ 1 gallon water (for each person)
- ❏ 1 jar peanut butter
- ❏ 1 large can juice (for each person)
- ❏ 1 can meat (for each person)
- ❏ Hand-operated can opener
- ❏ Permanent marking pen
- ❏ Pet food, diapers, and baby food, if needed

To Do:

- ❏ Find out what kinds of disasters can happen in your area. The easiest way to do this is to talk to your local emergency management agency, but you can also research local history at the library or the local newspaper. This will help focus your preparedness activities by letting you know what threats are realistic and which are not.
- ❏ Date each perishable item using a marking pen.

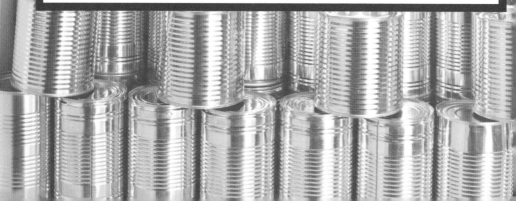

Project 1:
Bug out Bag (BOB)

Personally, it would take a very severe reason for me to evacuate or "bug out" from my home in the first place. Leaving the house would entail me having to leave many of my in-place systems and make me more vulnerable to outlaws and well-meaning (and not so well-meaning) bureaucrats.

However, just because I don't *want* to evacuate from my homestead doesn't mean I won't *have* to evacuate. I don't want any kind of disaster to befall my family, but measuring risk says I should be prepared "just in case." This leads me to the subject of disaster evacuation kits.

Any prepper or interested party with access to the Internet has probably noticed the love of acronyms as they relate to kits and gear. You have BOB, INCH, GOOD, GHB, EDC, IFAK, 72-hour kits, and 1st, 2nd, and 3rd line gear. The confusion just piles on.

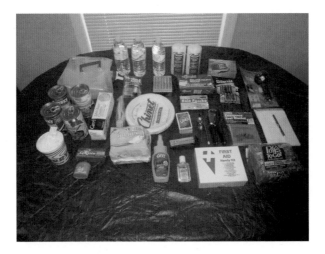

The reality is, it's pretty simple: It's all related to the things you need to survive under different scenarios. The concept of a 72-hour kit comes from the US military and is based on the fact that American soldiers are resupplied so often that they only need to be self-sufficient for three days at a time. This level is what the US government recommends for all citizens, because in the event of a federally declared disaster it will take FEMA approximately three days to get a supply system organized to provide relief. A 72-hour kit should have basic cooking, lighting, shelter, water, and food to survive for three days.

EDC, or "everyday carry," means the things you have on your body every day. BOB, bob, or B.o.B means "Bug Out Bag." A BOB is a small bag that is basically a portable 72-hour kit. The idea is that if a fire or something broke out and you had to leave *right now*, you can throw on your shoes, grab your BOB, and have whatever essential medicines, food, and clothes you would need. A good idea is to have copies of vital records in your BOB (project 1), so that you won't lose them if you don't have time to dig around in your filing cabinet.

A GHB, or "Get Home Bag," is practically the same as a BOB, but philosophically the opposite. A GHB is a portable kit containing the essentials you would need if you had to find an alternate route home if disaster struck while you were away from home. I keep a GHB in my vehicle, as well as my wife's. Due to the nature of cars, my GHB is actually a box that has a lot of stuff for light repairs, minimalist camping, and a walk home. Space and weight are not issues in the car, so I have things in my box that I can pick through to make a bag that best fits my situation.

Many people keep firearms in their GHBs and I understand that; however, if you have an assault rifle or other long arm and change into a multi-cam "uniform," you're going to attract unwanted attention. Consider a more concealable approach to defensive weaponry. In a disaster I want to blend in until I have to stand out.

A GOOD bag, or Get out of Dodge bag, is a larger BOB, but still small enough to carry. It's pretty much interchangeable with a BOB, just larger in scope. Some preppers have GOOD trailers or GOOD vehicles that are pre-packed. I use big plastic totes with a color code system.

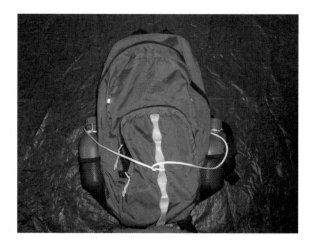

An INCH bag stands for "I'm Never Coming Home." It's more of a Mad Max/*The Road*/*The Postman* type problem where you have to take what you can carry, but all you own is what you take. My INCH bag would contain everything in my GOOD kit, plus extras like my hand-reloading press, more tools, and some small reference materials.

IFAK is an "individual first aid kit," also known as an "improved first aid kit" depending on the branch of service. This individual kit is part of a new military soldier initiative. It's a one-pound kit that addresses major blood loss and airway distress.

Line gear is also a military concept and centers around the gear you would need to complete a mission. It's not exactly applicable to citizen preppers, but it is related.

1st line gear is your EDC and focuses on what you would carry on your person. This would include your clothing, knife, weapon and, maybe a small survival and first aid kit.

2nd line gear is your "fighting load," which for me fits in a messenger bag. In this bag I can carry items like a flashlight, a hand-held radio, batteries, and calorie-dense energy bars. It also can go with me almost everywhere and gives me more capability without sacrificing a lot of maneuverability.

3rd line gear is your pack—sustainment items you need for a longer term. You're not going to fight wearing your rucksack; you would drop it and depend on your 1st and 2nd line gear during the fight and then go back and get your pack to refill your empty magazines.

It doesn't matter if you use the "proper" terms; just organize your gear to suit your needs. As long as you understand what you're doing and why you're doing it, you are light years ahead of guys that follow the conventional prepper wisdom and build kits based upon what some Internet guru wrote in a list.

It is important that you take some time to develop a plan that fits into your personal situation. All things being equal, less gear that you can use well and have on you is better than lots of gear you cannot use and do not carry.

That being said, today's project is to look around the house and assemble a small 72-hour kit to get you by until you finish your incremental disaster kit. Put in this kit everything you would need to survive 72 hours using the contents of this kit alone. Then schedule a weekend to try it out. Turn off the power and the water and see exactly how hard it is. This will show you the weaknesses of your kit, while putting you in a situation that could happen after a large winter storm or other natural disaster.

Week 2 Shopping List

To Buy:

- ❏ Heavy cotton or hemp rope
- ❏ Duct tape
- ❏ 2 flashlights with batteries
- ❏ Matches in waterproof container
- ❏ A leash or carrier for your pet

To Do:

- ❏ Complete a personal assessment of your needs and your resources for meeting your needs during a time of crisis. For example, if you have essential medical needs such as an oxygen concentrator, how would you power it? If you have a generator to do so, do you also have fuel?

Project 2:
Bug out Binder

Prepper or not, everybody should have a binder of important documents. After Hurricanes Katrina and Gustav I became aware of the difficulty many evacuees were having in relocating and becoming employed. You see, many of the Gulf Coast evacuees did not have their identity documents on them when they were forced to leave their homes.

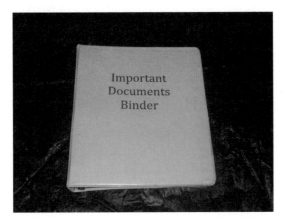

You may not have to evacuate due to a natural disaster, but everyone is at risk of a house fire, or just needing to be able to find important documents in a hurry.

It is very simple to buy a binder and some plastic sheet protectors to build a file that contains:

- Birth certificates
- Social Security cards
- Immunization records
- Diplomas
- Marriage/divorce documents
- Medical records/lists of needed prescriptions
- Insurance paperwork

- Mortgage documents
- Passports
- Retirement accounts

Additionally, I like scanning those documents and putting copies on a thumb drive and CD. They do not hold the same legal weight as an original copy, but they do help.

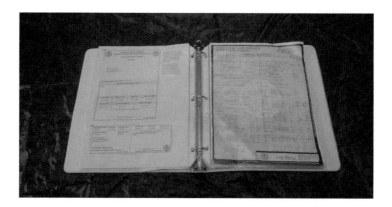

Because of the simplicity, the importance, and the likelihood of use, this is one of the very first steps a person should take to becoming prepared. Probably the only thing more important would be to sit down and discuss with your family what your concerns are and what threats you think are the most likely to impact your area and your family.

Week 3 Shopping List

To Buy:

- ❏ 1 gallon water (for each person)
- ❏ 1 can meat (for each person)
- ❏ 1 can fruit (for each person)
- ❏ Feminine hygiene supplies
- ❏ Paper and pencil
- ❏ Map of the area
- ❏ Aspirin or nonaspirin pain reliever
- ❏ Laxative
- ❏ 1 gallon of water for each pet

To Do:

- ❏ Create a personal support network that can help you identify and obtain the resources you will need to cope effectively with disaster.

Project 3: Water Storage

As a prepper, it's easy to get tunnel vision, focusing on storing food, learning skills, and acquiring gear. I find that there's a tendency to forget about the most basic needs because they are always there in the background.

The most overlooked resource is water. For pure survival water is second only to oxygen. We can only last a few hours to a few days without it, yet not many people store it in any quantity.

FEMA and the Red Cross have long suggested storing 1 gallon per person in your household per day for three days, but that is not enough. That small amount is going to be used up quickly in just drinking and cooking.

This project focuses on water storage to meet the base amount of water in your house to fulfill the ready.gov ideal of 72 hours.

The first thing you're going to need is something to store your water in. I use 5-gallon jerry cans. I like them because they are a good trade-off between size and capacity. However, many people I know use 2-liter soda bottles since they are a lot easier to carry, even if they are not as sturdy.

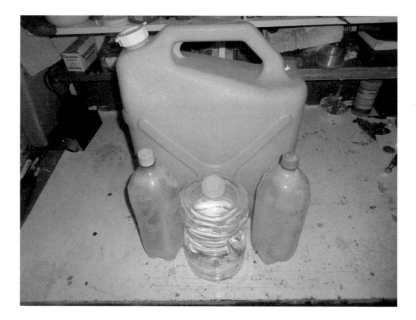

Do not become tempted and try to use milk jugs, as it is impossible to clean out the milk residue and it becomes a breeding ground for bacteria. Whatever you use, ensure it is food grade, clean, and able to be sealed.

Fill your container with clean water, the purer the better. Add bleach. FEMA guidelines recommend 1 teaspoon of nonscented bleach per quart of water. The bleach and water mix should smell slightly of chlorine. It's safe, since the chlorine loses its effectiveness over time and will eventually dissipate (just like the chlorine in your drinking water). However, since the container is sealed, the chlorine kills any pathogens in the water, and new bugs cannot contaminate the water.

Take precautions when filling and capping; make sure you don't contaminate the container with your hands.

Store your water in a cool, dry place, out of direct sunlight. This not only protects the plastic but also keeps algae from growing in the barrel if any survive.

This water does not have a shelf life, but some plastics can leach into the water, so twice a year (when I set the clock for daylight savings) I dump the water and refill the containers.

Week 4 Shopping List

To Buy:

- ❑ Patch kit and can of seal-in-air product for the tires of mobility aids such as cars, bikes, trailers, and wheelbarrows
- ❑ Signal flare
- ❑ Compass and local maps
- ❑ Extra medications or prescriptions marked "emergency use." There are several online resources to help you learn how to do this[1]

To Do:

- ❑ Develop a personal disaster plan.
- ❑ Give copies of the following lists to your network:
  - Emergency information list
  - Medical information list
  - Disability-related supplies and special equipment list
  - Personal disaster plan

[1]http://armageddonmedicine.net/
http://forecast.diabetes.org/supplies-aug2012
http://www.survivalblog.com/cgi-bin/mt5/mt-search.cgi?search=stockpiling+medications&IncludeBlogs=2&limit=20
http://theweekendprepper.com/health/prepping-and-prescription-drugs/

Project 4:
Tin Can Stove

In this project we are going to show you how to make a tin can stove; this type of stove has been around about as long as tin cans have been created, but it reached its peak of popularity during the Great Depression. Now its popularity is mostly with frugal backpackers and Girl Scouts.

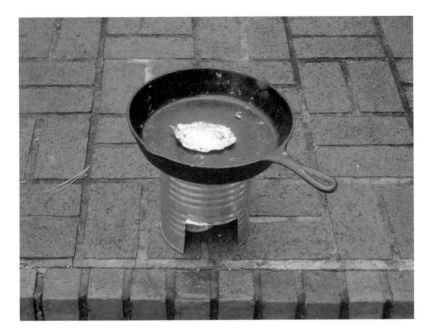

Personally, I feel that this stove has some pretty severe limitations: it's extremely hot, has little in the way of regulating heat, and its heating surface is small. However, as a way to begin to find new ways of using old things, upcycling, or making a MacGyverism, this stove is a good way of exercising your mind.

Materials:

- #10 can (empty, of course)
- Multiple tuna cans (also empty)

- Cardboard (lots of strips as wide as the tuna can is tall, you'll need a lot more strips than you think)
- Paraffin wax blocks
- Wick

Tools:

- Tin snips
- Can opener
- Double boiler
- Matches
- Razor or study scissors for cutting cardboard
- Gloves and other appropriate safety equipment

Procedure for stove:

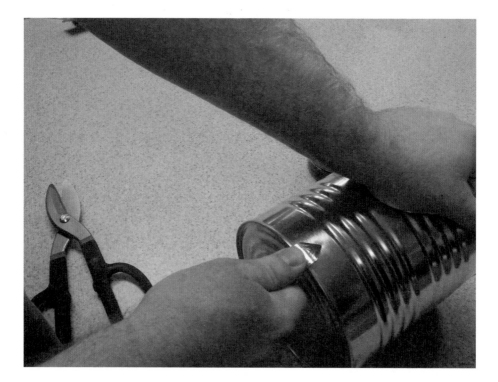

- Using a can opener, punch air holes around closed end of can. (Don't punch any air holes in the side you will have toward you, or smoke will blow in your direction.)

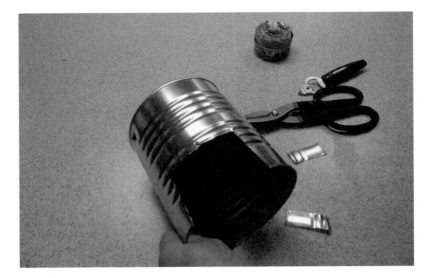

- Using tin snips cut a rectangle opening at open end of can, large enough to allow a burning tuna can to be pushed into, and pulled out of, the stove.
- Optional: use a metal coat hanger to fashion a damper on the stove opening using the scrap metal from cutting your opening.

Procedure for tuna can burner:

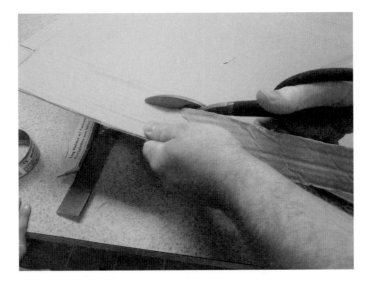

- Cut long cardboard strips as wide as your tuna can is tall.
- Tightly roll the strips into a small spiral.

- A piece of cotton wick inserted into the center of the cardboard helps in lighting the burner later.
- If you need to add more strips, overlap the end of the strip coming off the spiral with a new piece of cardboard so that it stays together on the roll.

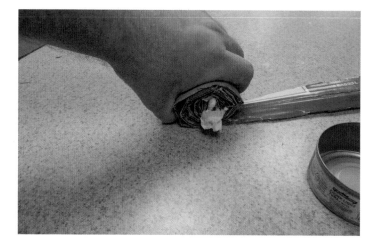

- Insert the spiral into the tuna can. This works best if the spiral is slightly larger than the can so that you must force it to fit. The more corrugated cardboard you can force into the can, the less wax you will need and the longer and hotter the fire will burn.

If needed, you can force additional cardboard strips between the can and the spiral of cardboard. This is not easy, but it makes everything work better later.

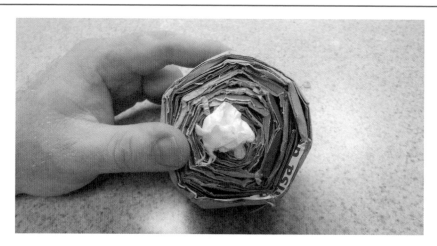

- Once you have made as many burners as your hands can stand (I can make about 6 before my arthritis makes me stop), melt the wax using a double boiler.

You should never heat wax over a direct source of heat, as it may flame up. If you do not have a double boiler, use a large pot of water with a smaller pot nested inside. The wax is placed in the small pot and is melted by the regulated heat of the water instead of the heat from the stove eye. This is much safer.

- Once the wax is melted, line the tuna cans up side by side and carefully fill them with wax. It takes a surprising amount of wax to fill the cans, especially if you did not fully pack the cans with cardboard.
- Let wax cool.

Procedure for using stove:

- Only use this stove outdoors, as it burns hot and with a lot of smoke.
- Place the stove on a surface that will not burn or be damaged by high heat.
- Light the tuna can burner and as soon as it flames place it inside the stove.
- It will only take a few seconds for the closed end of the can to reach cooking temperature, so don't touch it once the burner is inside (I learned this the hard way).
- Using a skillet is best, but you can cook things like hamburgers directly on the stove. It is too hot to cook things like eggs.
- Once cooking is complete, you can remove the stove and extinguish the burner.

I flip the burner upside down and smother the flame so I can reuse the can, but you could smother it with dirt. Don't douse it with water, or the hot wax may explode with some force and burn you.

Week 5 Shopping List

To Buy:

- ❏ 1 gallon water (for each person)
- ❏ 1 can meat (for each person)
- ❏ 1 can fruit (for each person)
- ❏ 1 can vegetables (for each person)
- ❏ 2 rolls toilet paper
- ❏ Extra toothbrush
- ❏ Travel-size toothpaste
- ❏ Special food for special diets, if needed

To Do:

- ❏ Make a floor plan of your home including primary escape routes.
- ❏ Identify safe places to go to in case of fire, earthquake, tornado, hurricane, and flood.
- ❏ Practice a fire drill, tornado drill, and earthquake drill with your network.

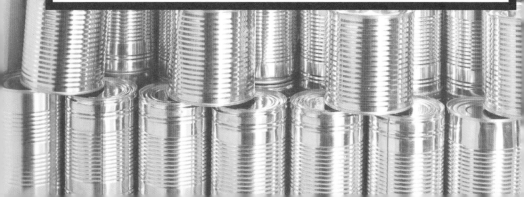

Project 5:
Mylar Bag Clamp

As I get more involved with personal disaster preparation and I store more dry bulk foods, I keep looking for ways to make what I am doing simpler and easier while still being cost effective. I have been searching for a solution to holding a full Mylar bag over the edge of a board while I try to juggle the bag, the iron, and the board without dumping everything, burning myself, or taking so long with the seal that I exhaust the absorbers.

This is a cheap and easy solution that holds your bags shut and allows you to make a strong seal using an iron.

All this clamp consists of is two 2x4 scraps and a hinge. On each board, I cut at a 45-degree angle along one of the long sides to allow a sharper area for sealing.

Since I sealed both 1- and 5-gallon Mylar bags, I cut the 2x4 into two sections that were a little longer than the open end of a 5-gallon Mylar bag. Using a simple hinge from my scrap box I connected the two 2x4 sections together.

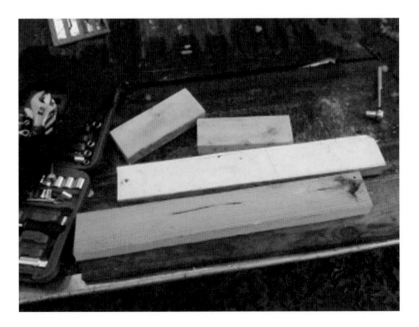

By clamping the open ends of the boards together, it holds the bag, which makes it *much* easier to iron. By facing the mitered edges of the board together, the "sharp" point also makes a crisp seal.

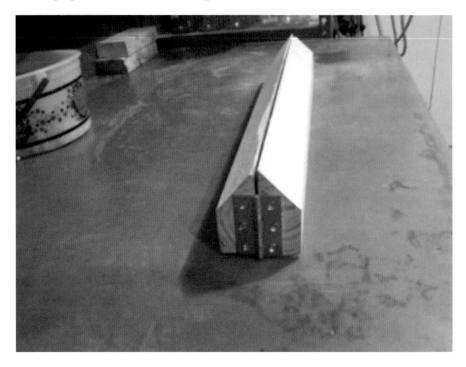

Since I made the boards longer than needed, later I plan on drilling a small hole between the two boards, so that I can insert a vacuum sealer hose inside the bag and can partially evacuate the air before sealing so that I can use a smaller and less expensive O_2 absorber.

Week 6 Shopping List

To Buy:

- ❏ Sterile adhesive bandages in assorted sizes
- ❏ Safety pins
- ❏ Adhesive tape
- ❏ Latex gloves
- ❏ Sunscreen
- ❏ Gauze pads
- ❏ Sterile roller bandages
- ❏ Extra hearing aid batteries, if needed

To Do:

- ❏ Check with your child's day care center or school to find out about their disaster plans.
- ❏ Ask your local emergency management office if emergency transportation services are available in case of evacuation.

Project 6:
Bulk Food Storage Using Mylar Bags

There are many reasons to store bulk food. Bulk food is cheaper, and when you buy in bulk you insulate yourself from rising food costs. Bulk food storage is the backbone of long-term emergency preparedness.

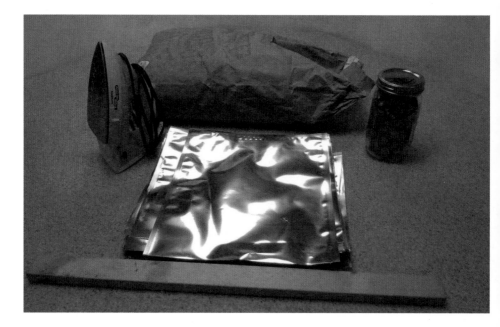

Packing and repacking bulk food into Mylar bags is one of the first skills most new preppers acquire. For this reason there are a lot of resellers that buy packing supplies and then repackage them at a profit. In my experience finding the best suppliers of both food and supplies is harder than the actual work of packing it.

I prefer to pack my food in 1-gallon bags because it is easier to use 1 gallon of food at a time than it is to use 5. Also, I can put several 1-gallon bags containing a variety of foods in a single 5-gallon bucket. I don't get as much in a bucket, but in the event I have to leave quickly and only have room for one or two buckets I don't risk as much. Typically I pack rice, wheat, sugar, and salt in the same bucket. I have many more options if I am eating out of a bucket like this than if I only had a bucket of wheat or salt.

Packaging this way helps if I want to provide charity, because I can give a single bucket at a time that contains multiple food items rather than a 5-gallon bucket of wheat berries.

The 1-gallon bags I use are 7 mil in thickness. This is the same thickness as an MRE retort package, but it is not the same exact material. I may use a thinner bag, but I do not use bags that are thinner than 5 mil, because I feel anything thinner is too flimsy to trust.

Oxygen absorbers are also needed. Normally they come in bulk packaged in a plastic vacuum seal bag. You need to be ready to use them, because as soon as the absorbers are exposed to air they begin working in a nonreversible process. Once they absorb the amount they are rated for they will not absorb any more oxygen.

Typically I pack everything, heat up the sealer, and have a mason jar ready to repack any unused absorbers. I open the pack and quickly insert the absorbers and seal everything up as quickly as possible to prevent waste.

The O_2 absorbers are typically labeled by amount of O_2 absorbed in cubic centimeters. The most common are 30 cc absorbers. To properly use them you need to calculate the size of the container and the density of what is to be

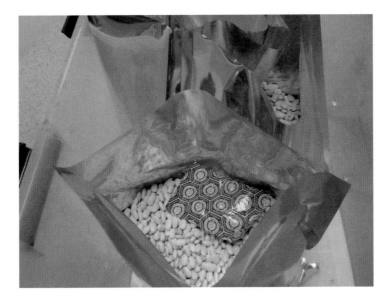

packed. Due to the grain size, there is a lot more air trapped in a gallon bag of potato chips than there is in a gallon bag of sugar.

Calculating amount of O_2 absorber needed:

First you need to know how many cubic centimeters of space are in your container. A gallon container is approximately 3785 cc. A #10 can is slightly smaller—most commonly .82 gallons for about 3104 cc of space. If you know that 1 cubic centimeter = 0.001 liters and 1 cubic centimeter = 0.00422675284 US cups you can calculate how many cc are in any container.

Next we need to know how much of that cc will be O_2 if it is empty. Only a percentage of the gas in our atmosphere is oxygen. Most of our air is nitrogen. Since nitrogen is inert we only have to worry about the 21 percent of the atmosphere that is O_2. To find out how much O_2 is in a container, multiply the cc size of the container by 21 percent.

As an example, to calculate the amount of oxygen sitting inside a 1-liter jug, you would need to multiply the 1000 cc of air by 20.95 percent and you would find that there is approximately 210 cc of oxygen inside the empty bottle.

But you are not storing an empty bottle, you're putting food in there, so you need to calculate how much space resides inside the spaces in between the food particles. If you were to fill your jug to the brim with dried macaroni, and then measure the amount of water, you could then see how much space was left in the voids of the macaroni shapes.

In a liter (1000 cc) of macaroni only approximately 495 cc is actually macaroni. This means there is approximately 505 cc of air sharing space with the macaroni inside the can. Multiply 505 by the 21 percent of O_2 in the air and you get 106.

This means to safely remove all the O_2 from a liter of macaroni you would need 150 cc of absorber (because the smallest absorber is 50 cc).

Procedure:

- Get bags set up. If using 5-gallon bags, place inside buckets; if using 1-gallon bags, I like to place them in a large plastic tote to avoid spillage.
- Fill bags. I use a quart jar as a scoop so that I can ensure I get an even amount of food in each bag.
- Heat iron or impulse sealer.
- Open O_2 absorbers and quickly put the required amount in each container, dump the rest in mason jars, and seal.

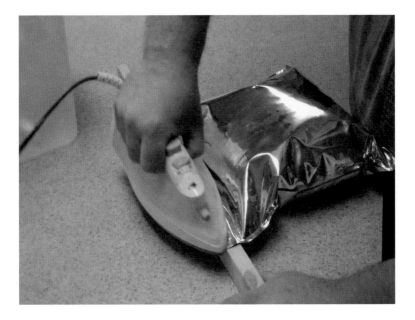

- Seal each bag, either using an impulse sealer, an iron and the bag clamp from the previous project, or the edge of a board.
- Make sure the bag is held tightly and the sealed edge is smooth. Do not overheat the bag; an iron on medium to medium-low works best. I prefer

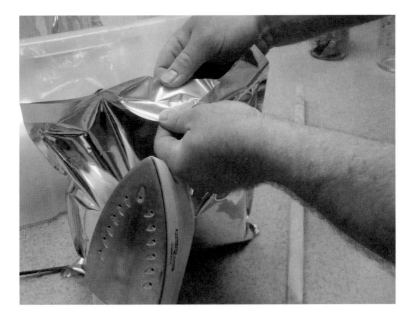

to make two small lines of seal, but some like a wider seal. What matters is that the seal is airtight.

- After each bag is sealed, check for leaks. I normally just turn the bags upside down over the plastic tub and shake.
- If you have sealed grains, beans, or any other item that may have insects, freeze them for at least 72 hours to kill any bugs. Typically, I rotate the bags into the freezer twice to ensure that I kill any insects and that any larva has time to hatch and be killed in the second freeze.
- Store in a cool, dark place away from humidity, and inside some sort of protective container. I use stackable plastic tubs, but if you have a rodent problem, metal garbage cans (new) work well.

Week 7 Shopping List

To Buy:

- ❑ 1 gallon water (for each person)
- ❑ 1 can ready-to-eat soup (not concentrated; for each person)
- ❑ 1 can fruit (for each person)
- ❑ 1 can vegetables (for each person)
- ❑ Sewing kit
- ❑ Disinfectant
- ❑ Extra plastic baby bottles, formula, and diapers, if needed

To Do:

- ❑ Establish an out-of-town contact to call in case of emergency.
- ❑ Share this information with your network so they know whom to call.
- ❑ Make arrangements for your network to check on you immediately after an evacuation order or a disaster.

Project 7:
Mason Jar Vacuum Sealer

Today's project allows you to use your vacuum food sealer attachments to seal mason jars without needing electric power.

This only works with *dried* food, as no heat is involved. So if you try to use it to preserve jelly or any other wet pack product you are at risk for botulism or other food-borne illness.

This is a very simple project. All you need are some canning jar adapters for use with a common vacuum food sealer. At the time of this writing the adapters were less than $10 each. They are readily available online or in big-box stores in the kitchen supply aisle.

You will also need a hand brake bleeder kit from an auto supply store. These run about $30–$35. If you can, try to find one that uses lead-free brass. Food should not be able to be vacuumed up into the actual pump, but in the very rare chance it is, you don't want food coming in contact with anything alloyed with lead. You also want to buy this new. If you buy a used pump then you run a serious risk of contaminating your food with hydraulic fluid left over from its previous use.

Your brake bleeder kit should have a long, clear plastic tube to attach it to the canning adapter, but if it does not, then you may need some ¼-inch aquarium line.

To use the hand pump to vacuum seal mason jars, follow these instructions:

- Attach the air line from the pump to the jar adapter.
- Place a new canning jar lid (just the lid, not the ring and lid) on the jar.
- Loosely press the jar adapter over the lid and onto the screw threads of the jar.
- Pump until the vacuum gauge on the brake bleeder reads at least 20 mHg.
- Release the vacuum and gently remove the adapter; the lid should be stuck firmly to the jar because of the internal vacuum.
- Screw ring on jar to keep seal.

This is for foods that are dry (moisture + vacuum = botulism) and that do not need refrigeration. Spices, popcorn, and very dry jerky are all things I have used this for. It also works well for nonfood items like bullets or band-aids.

Week 8 Shopping List

To Buy:

- ❏ Scissors
- ❏ Tweezers
- ❏ Thermometer
- ❏ Liquid antibacterial hand soap
- ❏ Disposable hand wipes
- ❏ Sewing needles (a pack with multiple sizes works best)
- ❏ Petroleum jelly or other lubricant
- ❏ 2 tongue blades
- ❏ Extra eyeglasses, if needed. Put in first aid kit.

To Do:

- ❏ Place a pair of sturdy shoes and a flashlight by your bed so they are handy in an emergency.
- ❏ If blind, store a talking clock and one or more extra white canes.
- ❏ If blind, mark your disaster supplies in braille or with fluorescent tape.

Project 8:
Ceramic Drip Water Filter

Go out now and find sources of water in your area, but remember, this is a basic need, and a small creek in the back of the subdivision may not supply enough water for *everyone* in the subdivision that knows about it.

Although you should store at least a 72-hour supply (or more), you also need some method of water purification. I chose to showcase this one method as it is easy to create and cost effective. I ordered this ceramic filter from a company called Monolithic for under $30 and installed it in under 30 minutes.

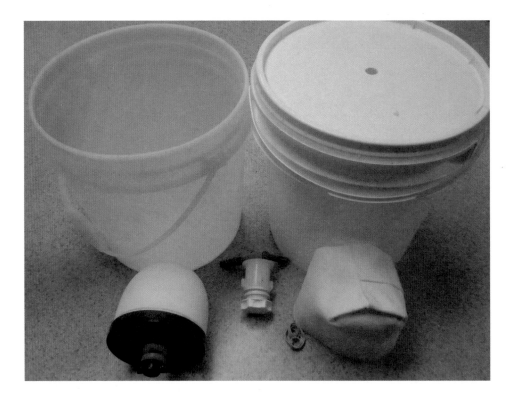

There are many ways of accomplishing the task. I used small plastic buckets from a local bakeshop, but you could use any food-safe container of any size as long the upper bucket can sit over the top of the lower container without crushing or falling over when filled.

Parts:

- Ceramic filter kit, containing:
- Filter
- Filter sock
- Spigot and gasket
- 2 food-grade buckets with lids

Tools:

- Drill with ½ and ¾ bits
- Small pipe wrench

Procedure:

- Mark center of one lid and center of bottom of one bucket. These marks must line up.

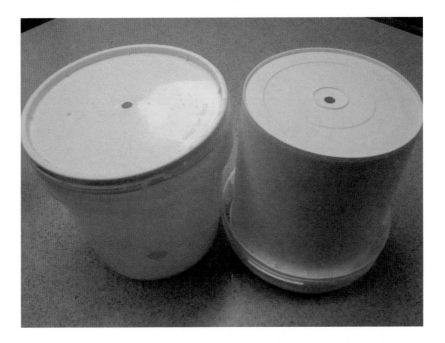

- Drill a ½-inch hole through the bottom of the bucket.
- Place bucket over the lid and verify the mark on the lid is in the center of the hole you drilled in the bucket.
- Drill hole through lid.
- Push filter nozzle through the hole in bucket and through the top of the lid. It should be a tight fit.
- Insert the gasket over the filter stem sticking out from the lid.
- Tighten wing nut on the stem until it is tight.

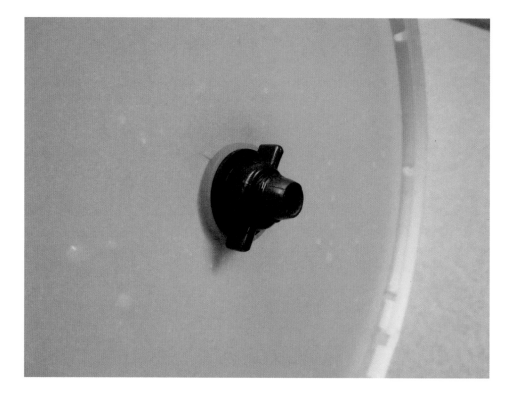

- Check for leaks. It is *vital* not to have any leaks into the bottom bucket or contaminated water will flow into it and recontaminate the clean water.
- Now the bucket containing the filter should be attached to the lid for the bottom bucket.
- Locate where you want to install the spigot on the bottom bucket. You want it anywhere from 1¼ to 2 inches from the bottom of the bucket so it won't rub on the countertop or table you keep it on.
- Drill a ¾-inch hole for the spigot.

- Place one washer on the spigot, flat side toward the valve on the spigot, and insert the spigot into the hole you drilled in the bottom container. After the spigot is put through the container, place the second washer onto the threaded portion of the spigot (angled side toward the wall of the bucket), place the hex head nut on the threads, and begin to screw on the nut.

You may turn the spigot instead of the nut if you wish. Do this until the nut becomes difficult to turn.

- Straighten the spigot so the handle is parallel to the bottom of the bucket. Finish tightening the nut so you have a watertight connection.
- Fill your container about half full with water and check for leaks.

If a leak is detected, tighten the nut on the spigot some more. Continue this action until no more leaks are detected.

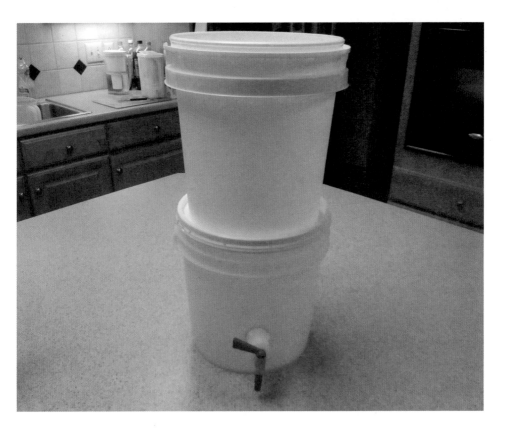

Sanitize the buckets:

Before inserting or using the filter system it is recommended to sanitize the containers with a diluted solution of bleach and water.

One teaspoon of bleach mixed with 1 gallon of water will do the job nicely. Wipe down the outside and the inside of each bucket with the bleach solution. Let stand for about 5 minutes, then wipe off with a dry paper or cloth towel.

Usage:

• Set on a level surface.
• Fill the top bucket with water.
• During the first use it can take up to several hours for the water to start flowing into the bottom container.
• As water is removed from the bottom container you may add that same amount of water to the top container, which will always keep your drinking water full.

Flow Rate:

It can take up to 36 hours for the flow rate to reach its maximum output. This is about 1–2 gallons per hour. The flow rate increases as the ceramic shell and the mixed charcoal media (inside the ceramic shell) become saturated with water.

Flow rate will decrease as the filter becomes clogged with use. You can clean with a Scotch Brite pad or something similar, but the use of any soap will destroy the filter.

Week 9 Shopping List

To Buy:

- ❏ 1 can ready-to-eat soup (for each person)
- ❏ Liquid dish soap
- ❏ Household chlorine bleach
- ❏ 1 box heavy-duty garbage bags with ties
- ❏ Antacid (for stomach upset)
- ❏ Saline solution and a contact lens case, if needed

To Do:

- ❏ Familiarize your network with any areas on your body where you have reduced sensation.
- ❏ Choose a signal with your network that indicates you are okay and have left the disaster site.
- ❏ If you have a communication disability, store a word or letter board in your disaster supplies kit.

Project 9:
Chicken Tractors

For those of you unfamiliar with the term, a chicken tractor is a cross between free-range chicken management and keeping them in a coop.

The idea is to have a small movable enclosure that allows the chickens to peck the ground freely, but still be confined and protected against predators.

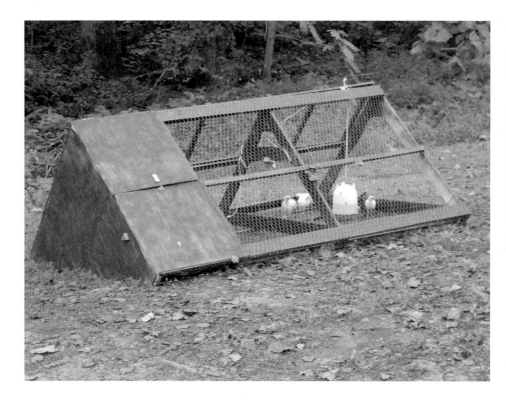

Because it's small the tractor can be moved every 7–10 days to prevent damage to the grass underneath.

We built a 6×12 A-frame and covered it on all sides but the bottom with hardware cloth. The bottom was covered in chicken wire to give better access to the grass.

In a tractor this size 5 or 6 chickens manage well, especially if you give them supplemental feed on top of the bugs and grass they find for themselves.

To make construction simple we built our chicken tractor like an A-frame. We cut most of the 1x4s into 4 foot sections with a 45-degree angle into one end.

Next, using glue, brads, and metal support plates used to make trusses, we built 4 sets of supports that were two of the 4-foot sections joined together to make a 90-degree angle.

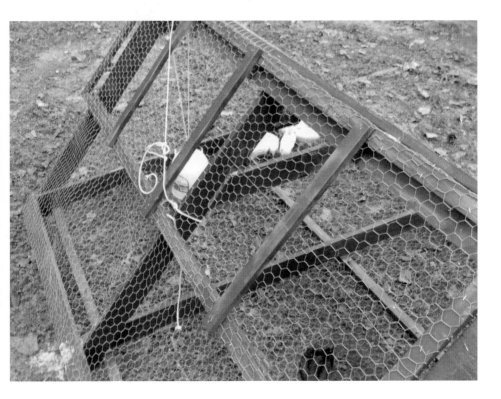

Once the 90-degree-angle sections were built, we attached them together by nailing them into 12 foot sections of 1x4 to make a frame.

Next a door was constructed out of 1x1 boards and chicken wire.

We cut two triangles into the plywood and then cut the remaining 4-foot piece into two 2-ft sections to make a "weather-proof" coop. A door was cut to allow the chickens inside, and a door was made on the outside to allow me to get the eggs.

Once the pullets got old enough to lay eggs, I made a nesting box out of an old milk crate I had scavenged.

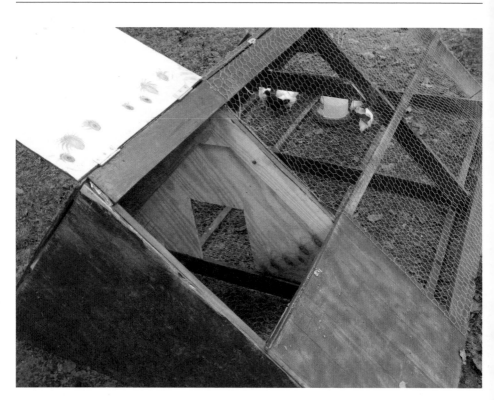

I bought all the materials new, (including tools) so we could not use any scrap. That being said, the cost for the 12-foot 1x4 boards, 8-foot 1x1 boards, hardware cloth, a roll of 4-ft chicken wire, one sheet of exterior-grade plywood sheathing, and the hardware cost about $200.

A commercial-built tractor of the same size starts at about $300 and up, so even factoring labor, it is still cheaper to build your own.

This was an easy enough project for two novices and took us about 10 hours.

I have read that some people also tractor rabbits, but when I tried it their manure piled up much quicker than the chickens', as chickens work it into the soil with their scratching.

Week 10 Shopping List

To Buy:

❏ Waterproof portable plastic container (with lid) for important papers
❏ Battery-powered radio
❏ Wrench needed to turn off utilities

To Do:

❏ Show your family the location of the gas meter and water meter shutoffs. Discuss when it is appropriate to turn off utilities.
❏ Attach a wrench next to the cutoff valve of each utility meter so it will be there when needed.
❏ Make photocopies of important papers and store safely.

Project 10:
Food Dehydration

Dehydrating vegetables allows them to last longer, take up less space, and weigh less. You can dehydrate your own vegetables with minimal processing or expense. Four bags of frozen vegetables dehydrate down to fit in a single mason jar; add water and they plump back up to almost the original size.

In an emergency, a pack filled with dehydrated food and access to water can be lifesavers.

The problem with dehydrating vegetables is that some vegetables need additional processing, either by blanching or by adding acid or some other solution to keep them from oxidizing. If you have ever eaten an apple and looked with disgust at the brown spots, you have seen oxidization. By soaking or dipping your potato or apple slices in lemon juice you can prevent this unsightly discoloration.

Some vegetables, like corn or beans, need to be blanched before dehydrating. Blanching is an essential process for dehydrating or freezing any vegetable except onions, peppers, and mushrooms. To blanch vegetables, cut them into the size you need, briefly boil them until they are just cooked, and then quickly dip them in ice water to stop the cooking process. Blanching kills the enzymes in the vegetables so that they do not lose flavor or texture.

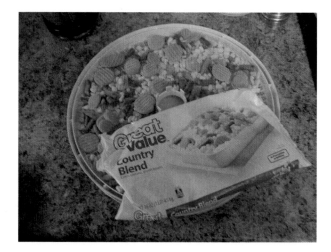

A tip for today's project is that if you dehydrate commercially frozen vegetables they are already prepared by blanching, so you can throw them straight from the bag into a single layer on your dehydrator.

Once the vegetables are dry, you can store them in mason jars or other air-tight container. It is important that there be *no* moisture allowed in the jar, as the dehydrated food will readily spoil if allowed to get wet. Botulism spores present on your vegetables can also begin to grow and produce their deadly toxin if they are vacuum sealed in a moist environment.

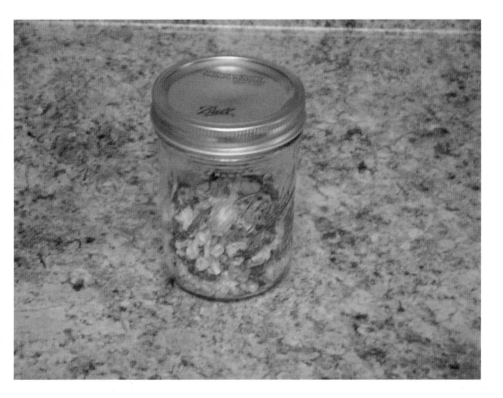

Make sure you have thoroughly dried your vegetables at 130 degrees. Beans, broccoli, carrots, cauliflower, corn, mushrooms, onions, peas, potatoes, tomatoes, and the like should be dried until brittle. Beets and sweet peppers can be dried until leathery.

The uses are almost limitless, if you have some imagination. Tomatoes can be ground after dehydrating, and then depending on the water added, can be used to make a paste, a sauce, or a soup. Paprika is a variety of pepper that is then dried and ground to make a spice. Feel free to experiment with your dehydrator and see what you like and what you don't.

At our house we cook a lot of stews, soups, and chili, which provides the perfect environment for cooking with dried vegetables.

Today's project is to dehydrate frozen store-bought vegetables in your oven so that you can experience using dried vegetables and decide for yourself if you want to work this skill into your disaster plan.

Procedure:

- Set your oven to a temperature lower than 200 degrees; in most ovens that would be the "warm" setting.
- Open your frozen vegetables and place on a cookie sheet. Personally I like using a pepper blend, but feel free to use whatever you prefer.
- Prop open the oven door slightly to allow moisture and water vapors to leave during the dehydration process.
- You can place a fan next to the oven to increase the airflow and temperature control.
- Leave alone for several hours (actual time may vary based upon moisture content, humidity, temperature, airflow, and elevation). Check every couple hours until it reaches desired level of dryness.
- Allow to cool before packing in airtight mason jars.
- Store in a cool, dry, dark location.

Week 11 Shopping List

To Buy:

- ❏ 1 large can juice (for each person)
- ❏ Large plastic food bags
- ❏ 1 box quick-energy snacks
- ❏ 3 rolls paper towels
- ❏ Medicine dropper

To Do:

- ❏ Test your smoke detector(s). Replace the battery in each detector that does not work.

Project 11:
Dehydrating Hamburger (aka Hamburger Rocks)

Dehydrated hamburger is commonly called "hamburger rocks" online. When you make some you will quickly learn how it got its name. Once the hamburger is cooked and dried it resembles really small dark brown gravel. The reason we make it is not to have small meat stones but because when stored under a

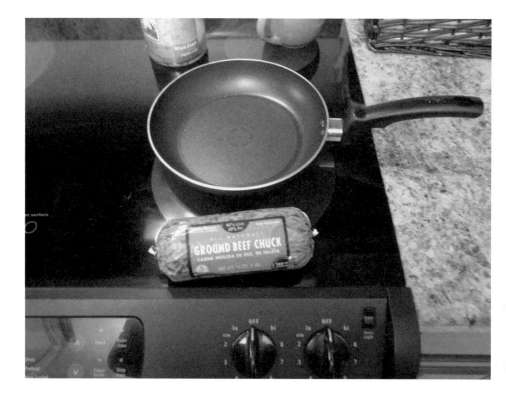

vacuum, and kept in a cool dry place, our hamburger rocks last much longer than fresh hamburger.

While nothing beats fresh meat, this ingredient works very well in any recipe that uses browned ground beef. I use it quite often in making chili, tacos, or spaghetti.

The recipe for rehydrating is subject to personal preference, but I find a 1:1 ratio of rocks to water works best (since I use it mostly in chili and lasagnas and allow the rocks to absorb juices during cooking). Most people prefer to rehydrate with more water and usually use 1 cup rocks to 2 cups boiling water and let it rehydrate prior to using it their recipes.

Now, be prepared to cry a little when you're done, as 5 or 6 pounds of ground meat will dehydrate away to a less than a quart jar of rocks, and you

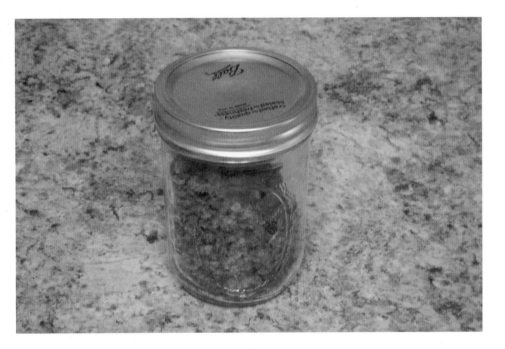

may think you wasted a lot of good meat. However, it is the decrease in size that is helpful for long-term storage, and the size decrease is fat and water, so you are not really losing anything you can't add back later.

The recipe is simple:

Instructions:

• Cook ground beef.
• Drain fat.

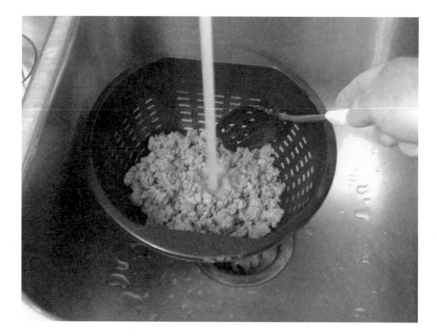

• Rinse meat in a colander to remove all fat.
• Recook to drive off water. Cook until steam stops.
• Dehydrate.

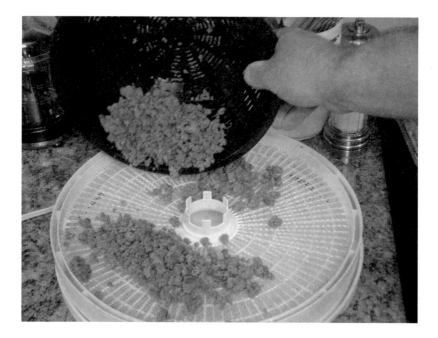

I use a dehydrator with a temperature setting and dry it at 160 degrees Fahrenheit for 8 hours.

You could use an oven by putting the beef on a roasting pan and putting in a 200-degree oven with the door open slightly, continually monitoring and stirring the beef until dry (though if you have completed the last project you may already know it's easier with a dehydrator).

Once it is dry, cool, and hard to the touch, vacuum seal in mason jars or bags.

Alternatively, while the rocks are still hot, you could "can" the hamburger rocks for long-term storage: preheat mason jars to 250 degrees Fahrenheit simmer the lids as usual, put the rocks into the jars while still hot, and then seal the jars. After 15 minutes or so the jars will cool and you will hear the jar lids "pop" as they seal in place. This is not my favorite method, but it is similar to a vacuum seal. However, be aware this method is not FDA approved and has not been scientifically evaluated to prevent botulism poisoning.

Vacuum-packed rocks, stored in a cool, dry, dark location, will last about 1 year before turning rancid.

Week 12 Shopping List

To Buy:

❏ Extra harness, leash, ID tags, and food for your service animal and/or pets
❏ Litter/pan
❏ Extra water
❏ Obtain current vaccinations and medical records for your animal(s)

To Do:

❏ Develop a pet care plan in case of disaster.
❏ Make photocopies of all vaccination records and put them in your disaster supplies kit.
❏ Put extra animal harness, leash, and identification tag(s) in your disaster supplies kit.

Project 12:
How to Make Dakin's Antiseptic Solution

Dakin's solution is an antiseptic solution containing sodium hypochlorite (common household bleach) and water. It was first developed during World War I to treat infected wounds.

Dakin's solution is obviously not the only antiseptic available. Several stronger germicidal solutions, such as those containing carbolic acid (phenol) or iodine, can be purchased and used to prevent infection.

Unfortunately, the stronger solutions either damage living cells or lose their potency in the presence of blood. Dakin's solution does neither. Additionally, its action as a solvent to dead cells hastens the separation of dead from living tissue.

Dakin's solution is easy to make and is prepared by passing chlorine into a solution of sodium hydroxide or sodium carbonate.

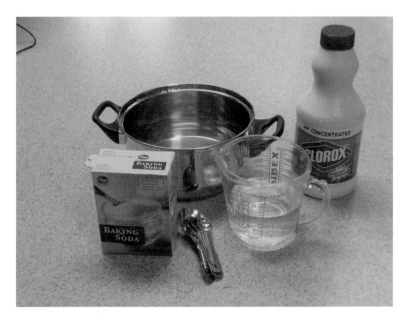

Unfortunately, the solution is unstable and cannot be stored more than a few days. Thirty days is the most you can expect if stored under the best conditions.

It is used by periodically flooding an entire wound surface with the solution. I have used this solution on myself, as well as on my animals. It does not sting or burn as much as you might expect, and is credited with saving thousands of lives during the Great War.

As always, I am not a doctor, and you should research anything you read so you are assured of its use and the accuracy of the material presented.

Precautions:

- Keep out of the reach of children.
- Do not swallow if used as a mouth wash.
- Do not use longer than 1 week.
- Obviously, do not use this solution if you are allergic to any of the ingredients.
- Stop use of the solution if your condition worsens, or a rash or any other reaction develops.

Call Your Doctor If You Have:

- Pain or burning sensation
- Rash or itching
- Redness of skin
- Swelling, hives, or blisters
- Signs or symptoms of wound infection

Storage:

Keep the solution stored at room temperature, tightly sealed, and away from light.

Cleanliness is very important to this procedure; sterilize everything, and keep your hands clean. Remember the maxim: you cannot sterilize what is not clean.

Equipment:

- Clean pan with lid

- Sterile measuring cup and spoons
- Sterile jar with sterile lid (see above)
- Clean pan with lid
- Sterile measuring cup and spoons
- Sterile jar with sterile lid (see above)

Procedure:

- Measure out 32 ounces (4 cups) of tap water. Boil water for 15 minutes with the lid on the pan. Remove from heat.

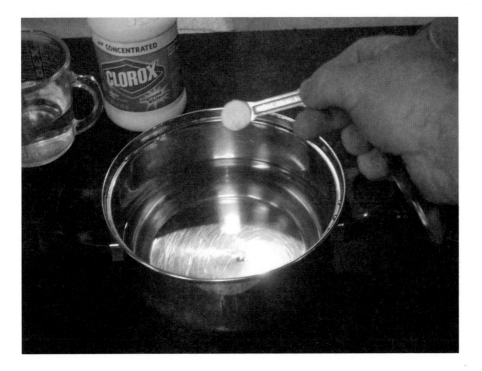

- Using a sterile measuring spoon, add ½ teaspoon baking soda to the boiled water.
- Place the solution in a sterile jar. Close it tightly with the sterile lid.
- Label the jar with the date and time you made the solution.

Throw away any unused portion 48 hours after opening. Unopened jars can be stored for 1 month after you have prepared them.

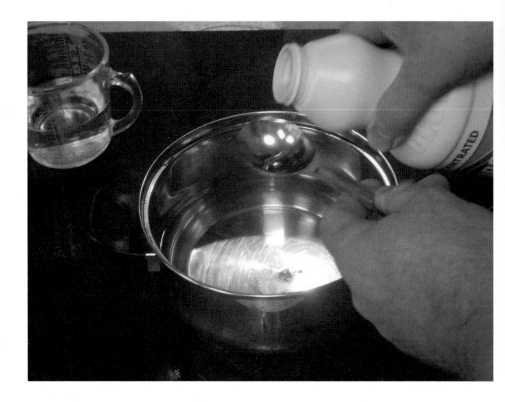

Strength of Solution is dependent on how much bleach to water. The following chart is for 32 ounces of water.

	Full Strength	½ Strength	¼ Strength	⅛ Strength
Bleach	3 oz.	3 tbsp. + ½ tsp.	1 tbsp. + 2 tsp.	2½ tsp.

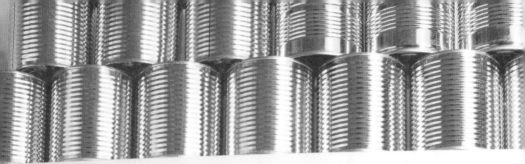

Week 13 Shopping List

To Buy:

- ❏ Whistle
- ❏ Pliers
- ❏ Screwdriver
- ❏ Hammer
- ❏ Perforated metal tape (sometimes called plumber's tape or strap iron)
- ❏ Crow bar

To Do:

- ❏ Take a first aid/CPR class.
- ❏ Arrange to have your water heater strapped to wall studs using perforated metal tape.

Project 13:
How to Make Sugardine Antiseptic Solution

Sugardine is an antiseptic that uses the antibacterial properties of both pure sugar and iodine to prevent and kill infections. It is primarily used to treat abscesses and thrush on the hooves of horses, but it can be used in many other

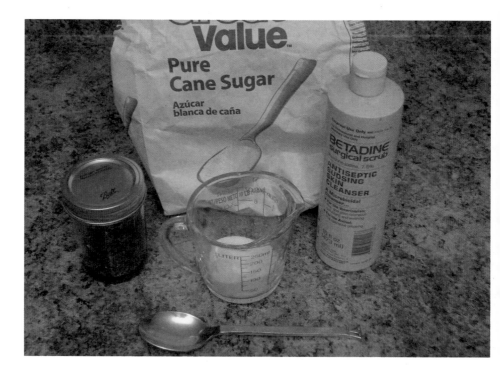

ways. As a side benefit to the prepper, it is cheap and easy to make as well as effective if used properly.

Although it is true that a diluted sugar solution will feed bacteria and mold, (that is how we get all sorts of alcoholic drinks), when sugar is highly concentrated it sucks the moisture right out of bacteria so that it cannot live.

Just think, have you ever had white table sugar grow any bacteria or fungus while it's just sitting out on your counter?

When you add the iodine to make a paste, the iodine provides not only a second line of defense but it also holds the sugar together so you can pack it around the wound. Just sprinkling sugar on the wound would not hold enough sugar to keep the blood and other fluids from diluting, so it would feed the infection instead of killing it.

Basically, if you have a soft-tissue wound like a cut, abscess, or burn, you would put the Sugardine on the wound and cover with a bandage. If the wound is leaking, you want to replace the sugar on a regular basis, as if it gets waterlogged, it will do more harm than good.

When making the Sugardine, it's best to start with an amount of sugar close to the amount of finished product you want and slowly add the Betadine or Povidone until you get the thick peanut butter texture. Otherwise, you will most likely use too much liquid and have to add sugar repeatedly until you end up with much more Sugardine than you intended.

Ingredients:

• Table sugar
• 10 percent povidone-iodine (or Betadine—but it is more expensive because it is a brand)

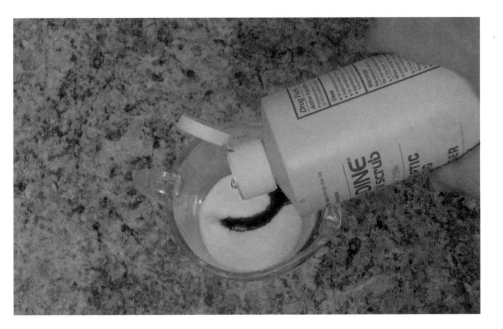

Procedure:

- Mix one part 10 percent povidone-iodine to two parts white sugar.
- Add more or less sugar to reach desired consistency; it should be like thick honey when all mixed together.
- Put the Sugardine in a container with a lid.

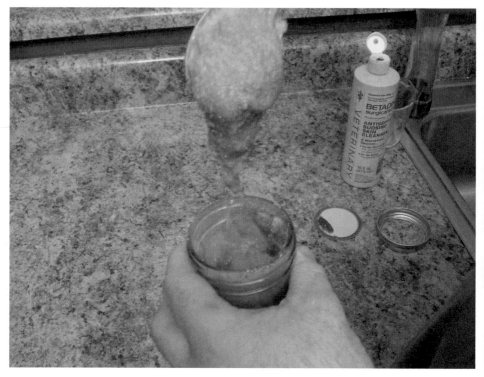

It Should be Thick and "Gloopy" like Peanut Butter

The mixture will need stirring now and then, but it will never go bad. I have some that is three years old, and although it is darker than it was originally, it is still usable.

Week 14 Shopping List

To Buy:

- ❏ 1 can fruit (for each person)
- ❏ 1 can meat (for each person)
- ❏ 1 can vegetables (for each person)
- ❏ 1 package eating utensils
- ❏ 1 package paper cups/plates

To Do:

- ❏ Make sure your network and neighbors know what help you may need in an emergency and how best to assist.
- ❏ Practice using alternate methods of evacuation with your network.

Project 14:
Clothes Washer from Plunger

In order to make a nonelectric washing machine, I bought a simple plunger from the local box store and drilled some small holes around the base to help keep the water from sudsing over, as well as to help push water through the clothing. I also unscrewed the short handle and replaced it with a mop handle so I don't have to bend over and work as hard. This also gives me more leverage.

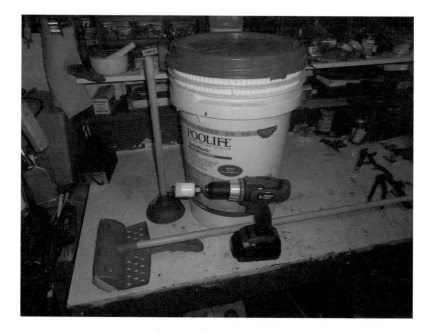

I cut a hole the size of the handle in the center of a tight-fitting bucket lid.

To wash, all I do is add a few articles of clothing to the bucket, about ¼ cup of my handy homemade liquid detergent, and about 1 ½ gallons of water to the bucket. Insert the plunger, and then lock on the lid.

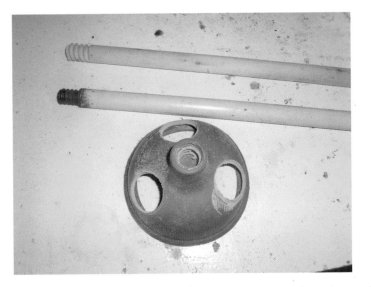

I push the plunger around the clothes for a minute or 5, then dump the dirty water, add clean rinse water, and repeat until the rinse water comes out clean.

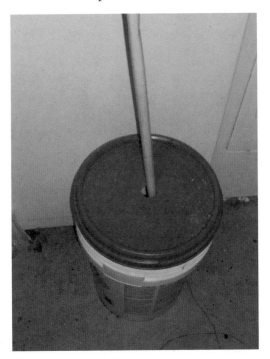

If you want you could add bluing to the rinse to whiten your clothes. I don't do this right now, but I have some just in case this becomes my primary method of washing clothes.

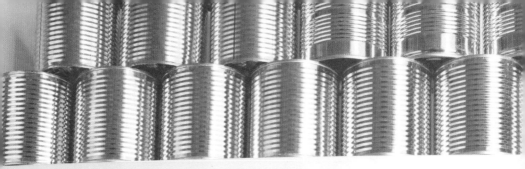

Week 15 Shopping List

To Buy:

- ❑ Extra flashlight batteries
- ❑ Extra battery for portable radio
- ❑ Assorted nails
- ❑ Wood screws
- ❑ Labels for your equipment and supplies

To Do:

- ❑ Make arrangements to bolt bookcases and cabinets to wall studs.
- ❑ Label equipment and attach instruction cards.

Project 15:
Turning Baking Soda to Washing Soda

While researching soap recipes, I kept finding recipes using washing soda, with warnings not to confuse it with baking soda. Since I believe that most warning labels are posted in response to someone getting hurt, I think it is important to explain the difference so that people have enough information to stay safe.

Here is the difference between them: Washing soda is sodium carbonate—two sodium atoms, a carbon atom, and three hydrogen atoms. Baking soda is sodium bicarbonate—the same ingredients, but with a hydrogen atom replacing one of the sodium atoms.

What that means to us is that their pH is different. Baking soda is about an 8 on the scale (7 being neutral), which makes it a weak base. Since most of our body fluids are around 7.4, baking soda is not that corrosive to our bodies.

Washing soda, on the other hand, is about an 11 on the scale, which means it is a relatively corrosive. As a matter of fact, it is far enough on the pH scale that it is not allowed to be labeled "nontoxic." You do not want to get this in your body.

But since washing soda is more base, it can neutralize more acid, so it's perfect for washing things like dirty diapers.

Washing soda (sodium carbonate) and baking soda (sodium bicarbonate) are not interchangeable in soap and other recipes. Unfortunately, it is not always easy to find washing soda at the big-box chain stores.

I have been looking for a way to get around this, and the solution was surprising simple.

Basically, the difference between baking soda and washing soda is water and carbon dioxide.

In the beginning portion of this project, we told you what molecules made up both baking and washing soda. If you add heat energy, baking soda breaks down. It releases steam (H_2O) and carbon dioxide (Co_2) from the soda, and what you have left is washing soda.

As a word of precaution, you don't want to do this in huge quantities, or with your face right over the pot—the carbon dioxide displaces oxygen and you could conceivably pass out or suffocate.

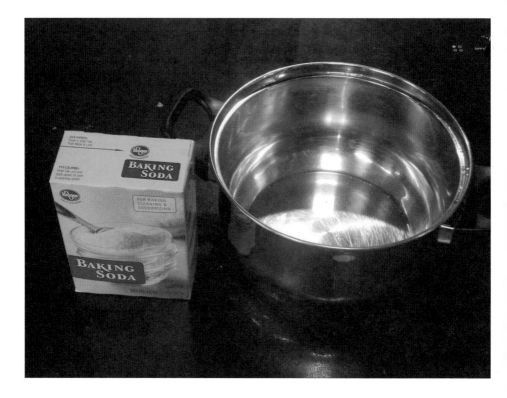

Here is the *very* simple procedure:

- Fill a wide baking dish with baking soda. (You can also do this on a stove-top.)
- Heat in the oven at 400 degrees until all the baking soda becomes washing soda.
- Occasionally mix it so that this process happens faster and more uniformly. (The process starts at about 140 degrees, but within reason the higher the heat, the faster the transformation.)

This takes about 45 minutes for a normal-sized box of baking soda—exact times depend on the container you use, the humidity in the air, and the heat.

The more spread out the soda is, the faster it transforms. However, overcooking is not an issue, so if you go for a couple hours it will be fine.

Once it is done, you will notice a difference between the two—baking soda is white, powdery, and will clump together. Washing soda is more gray, grainier, and duller.

If you did this over a stovetop, the baking soda will "boil" and erupt little steam geysers—which makes for a cool science demonstration if you have kids.

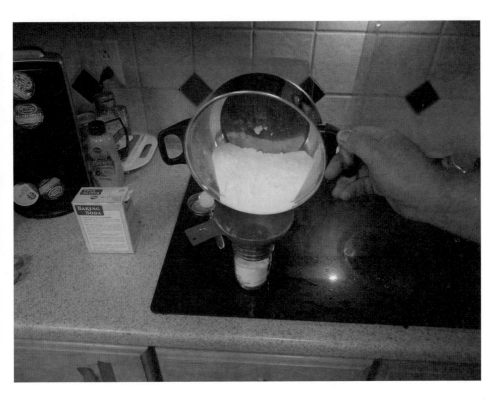

Store your washing soda in an airtight container away from moisture. Also, remember it is a stronger base and is not as safe as baking soda.

Week 16 Shopping List

To Buy:

- ❏ 1 can meat (for each person)
- ❏ 1 can vegetables (for each person)
- ❏ 1 box facial tissue
- ❏ 1 box quick-energy snacks
- ❏ Dried fruit/nuts

To Do:

- ❏ Find out if you have a neighborhood safety organization and join it.
- ❏ Develop a disaster supplies kit for your car or van.

Project 16: Liquid Laundry Soap

If you're going to be out growing food or camping or building skills, you're going to get your clothes dirty too. I know it's simple to go to the store and buy whatever laundry soap you like to buy, but something else I have learned about preppers is that they like to save money, and don't mind putting in some extra work to do so.

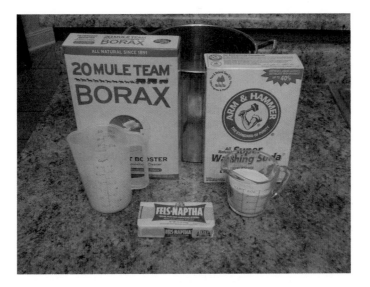

After calculating the costs of material this soap costs about 3 cents a load. Factoring in my time brings it to 10 cents a load. It's still cheaper than *any* liquid laundry soap on the market.

The best thing is that you can control the ingredients, so it works great for those with sensitive skin.

The only down-side is that it doesn't quite have the familiar texture you're used to; to me it looks a lot like pale green snot. But you have to trade off somewhere and in a comparison between a lumpy gooey soap for next to nothing and overly scented, expensive soap that has a consistent texture, I'm going to choose cheap.

Equipment:

- 5-gallon container
- Box or other grater
- Pot large enough to hold 6 cups of water
- Long stirring stick or spoon for 5-gallon container

Ingredients:

- ½ of a 5.5-ounce bar of Fels Naptha soap
- 1 cup 20 Mule Team Borax
- ½ cup Arm & Hammer Super Washing Soda
- Water

Procedure:

- Grate the soap into small slivers. Fels Naptha soap seems to work the best for me, but you could use any bar soap.
- Heat 5 cups of water in a large pot.
- As the water heats, gradually add the soap slivers. You do not want the water to boil, or the soapy water will bubble over. As the slivers melt, keep adding until all the soap is melted.

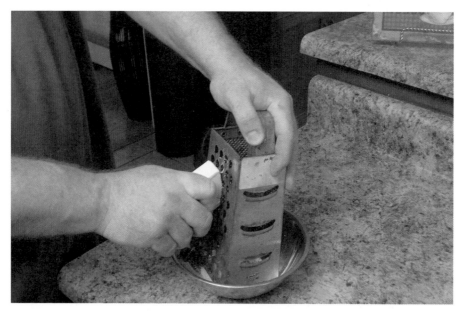

Warning: don't use your wife's favorite grater.

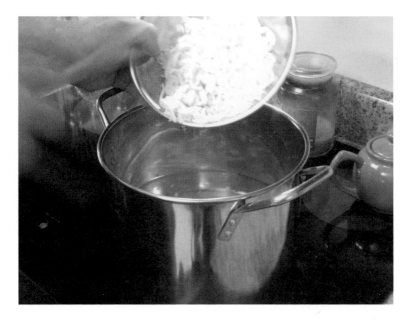

- Place 3 gallons of hot water into the 5-gallon container.
- Pour the melted soap mixture into the container of hot water. Stir.
- Add washing soda. Stir until the soda dissolves, and then add Borax. Stir until dissolved.

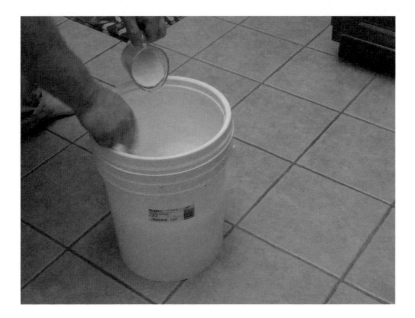

- To add fragrance, if desired, add a few drops of essential oils of your favorite scent.
- Cover the container and set it aside. Let it sit overnight so it can cool and gel. The detergent will not gel uniformly; it may appear watery and clumpy.

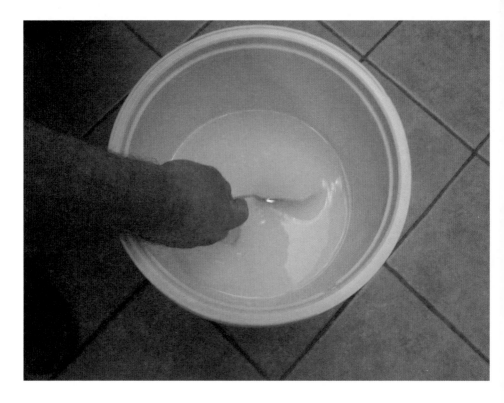

Week 17 Shopping List

To Buy:

- ❏ 1 box graham crackers
- ❏ Assorted plastic containers with lids
- ❏ Dry cereal
- ❏ Antidiarrheal medication
- ❏ Rubbing alcohol
- ❏ Antiseptic
- ❏ Syrup of ipecac and activated charcoal

To Do:

- ❏ Arrange for a friend or neighbor to help your children if you are not able to respond or are at work.

Project 17: Fuel-Efficient Rocket Stove

Being able to sustainably cook and heat is something that every prepper needs to plan for. It is not uncommon for modern homes to rely solely upon electricity for both. Today's project is a means to use twigs to create a very clean burning stove that provides a lot of heat without having to burn large amounts of wood.

A rocket stove is able to burn efficiently by using high temperature and a good air draft coming from the bottom of the stove. Once the basic premise is understood, these stoves can be quickly built from improvised materials at hand. In this project we will use a #10 can as the base, but I have seen commercially built stoves using 55-gallon drums, or even homebuilt stoves out of stovepipe and rock used to preserve food outdoors.

Equipment:
- Tin snips
- Hammer
- Pliers
- File
- Gloves
- Drill, punch, or nail
- Marker

Ingredients:
- Empty #10 can (sometimes you can get these for free from local restaurants, but I bought a bulk pack of chili beans to acquire this one)
- Four 10.5-ounce soup/vegetable can
- Insulation (perlite, sand, dirt, ash—basically any flame-resistant insulating material)

Procedure:

- Remove all labels from all the cans and clean cans well.
- Mark and cut hole in #10 can:
    - Use one of your cans to trace a circle onto the #10 can. It should be about ½ inch from the bottom of the #10 can.
    - Next drill, punch, or nail some access holes inside the drawn circle so that you can cut out the circle using your tin snips
    - Make sure a can (can B) is able to fit snugly in the hole.

- Mark and cut hole in the side of a soup can (can A):
    - This hole needs to be at the same height as the hole in the #10 can. It may be best to insert this can into the larger one and mark it through the hole in the #10 can.
    - Since this can needs to form an "elbow," make sure that can B can fit securely in the hole.

- Cut bottom off of soup can (can B) and fit as elbow:
    - If you can use a can opener, do so, but newer style cans make this harder, so you may need to use tin snips.

- Cut and fit the chimney from soup can (can C):
    - Slit can C from top to bottom.
    - Cut an arch at the bottom of the can, so it can sit on can B once the stove is assembled. Once assembled, can C must sit approximately ¼ inch below the edge of the #10 can.

- Cut a hole in the lid of the #10 can for the chimney.
    - Take a can and center it on the #10 can lid, trace the circle, and cut it out with tin snips.

- Assemble:
    - Set can A into the #10 can, ensuring that the open end of can A is facing up.
    - Push can B through the hole cut into the #10 can and into the hole cut into can A.
    - Can A should be centered into #10 can, with a portion of can B sticking out of the side of the #10 can.

- Push can C into the top of can B forming a chimney.

• Cut 8 slits ½ inch long vertically from the top of the #10 can.
• Fill with insulation material:

- Go slow, and from time to time gently shake or rap the #10 can so that the insulation settles. Take care not to disturb the assembly.

• Insert #10 can lid over chimney formed by can C:

- Press the lid down slightly.
- Secure the lid by bending every other tab formed by the ½-inch slits in the top of the #10 can. This should leave 4 tabs standing up to hold a cooking pot upright.
- The top of the chimney should be below the edge of the 4 upright tabs.

• Make a fuel shelf from a soup can (can D):

- With the remaining can (or a larger one), cut the can open lengthways and flatten it out.
- Cut a "t" shape into the can, with the long leg approximately the size of the width of the center of can B.
- Leave "wings" slightly larger to keep the shelf from being pushed into the stove.

• Start a fire:

- This stove will get hot! You are warned.
- Wad some paper or tinder, light it, and drop down the chimney.
- Push small twigs or other kindling-sized fuel into the stove through can B; it should sit on top of the shelf you just cut.
- Air will flow into the stove through the channel under the shelf.
- As the fuel burns, push it deeper into the stove so that it can fully combust.

Week 18 Shopping List

To Buy:

❏ "Child proof" latches or other fasteners for your cupboards
❏ Double-sided tape or hook-and-loop fasteners (such as Velcro®) to secure moveable objects
❏ Plastic bucket with tight lid
❏ Plastic sheeting

To Do:

❏ Arrange for someone to install latches on cupboards and secure moveable objects.
❏ Put away a blanket or sleeping bag for each household member.

Project 18:
Wheat Grinding

If you're going to store wheat, you need to be able to grind it. You really ought to consider buying a quality wheat grinder; however, if you are unwilling, or unable to do so there is a way you can grind wheat without a grinder.

Be aware that this has some serious disadvantages; it is not as easy as turning a crank (and that isn't easy either), it is louder, and the wheat is not ground as fine.

Today's project will not only show you how to grind wheat without a mill but also it will probably convince you that a mill is the best way to go.

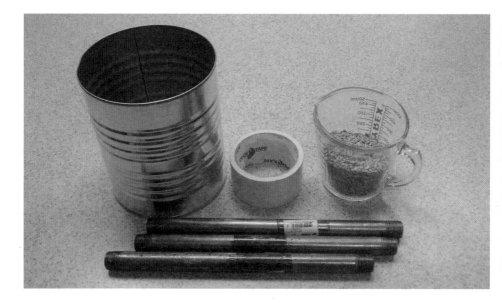

Grinding Wheat without a Mill:

Equipment:

- 90 inches of ¾ water pipe cut into three 30 inch lengths of pipe
- Empty #10 can or other small metal container

- Tape or sturdy string
- Whole wheat or dried corn

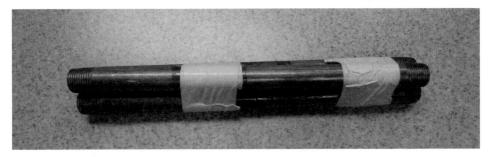

Procedure:

- Tape or otherwise bind the 3 pipes into a secure bundle so that their working ends are as even as possible and flat enough to sit evenly on a hard surface.
- Cut the top smoothly out of a large can. A #10 can is ideal. If you do not have a can, improvise something to keep grain together while pounding it.

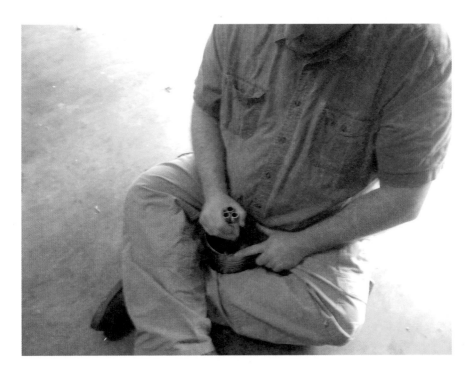

- Put clean, dry grain about 1 inch deep in bottom of the can.
- Place the can on a hard, smooth, solid surface, such as concrete.
- To pound the grain, sit with the can held between your feet. Move the bundle of pipes straight up and down about 3 inches, with a rapid stroke.
- To separate the pounded grain into fine meal, flour, coarse meal, and fine-cracked wheat, use a sieve made of window screen.
- To separate flour for feeding small children, place some pounded grain in an 18x18 inch piece of fine nylon net, gather the edges of the net together so as to hold the grain, and shake this bag-like container.

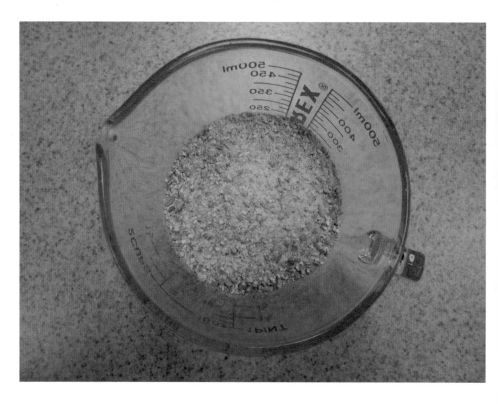

- To make flour fine enough for babies, pound fine meal and coarse flour still finer, and sieve it through a piece of cheesecloth or similar material.
- Buy a grain mill, the best you can afford.

Week 19 Shopping List

To Buy:

- ❏ 1 box quick-energy snacks
- ❏ Comfort foods (such as cookies or candy bars)
- ❏ Plastic wrap
- ❏ Aluminum foil
- ❏ Denture care items, if needed

To Do:

- ❏ Review your insurance coverage with your agent to be sure you are covered for the disasters that may occur in your area. Obtain additional coverage, as needed.
- ❏ Purchase and have installed an emergency escape ladder for upper-story windows, if needed.

Project 19: Wheat Berry Blender Pancakes

Of all the food storage recipes I have learned to make, this one is my wife's favorite. It's also a winner on a weekend morning, because it's easy, cheap, and gets me points for when I plan on spending the day on a project.

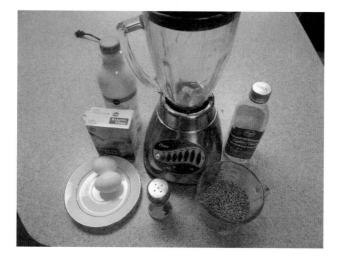

Ingredients:

- 1 cup milk (translation for powdered milk is 3 tbsp. milk and 1 cup water)
- 1 cup wheat berries
- 2 eggs (2 tbsp. powdered eggs, ¼ cup water)
- 2 tbsp. baking powder
- 1½ tbsp. salt
- 2 tbsp. oil
- 2 tbsp. honey or sugar

If you really want a healthy treat, use buttermilk and let the wheat berries soak in it overnight. The acid in the milk helps break up the wheat making it more digestible (it also makes it taste better).

Add the wheat and milk in the blender and pulse until the wheat turns to batter. Add the other ingredients and pulse for a couple minutes more. This works because the blender is made to mix wet ingredients and so it works best with liquids. After every couple pancakes pulse the batter for a second or two to keep everything mixed.

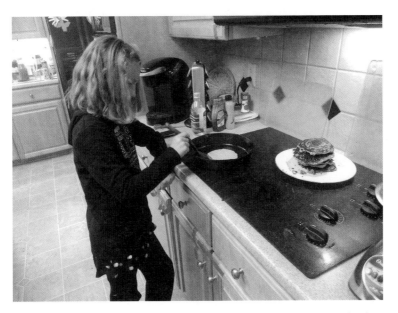

(They are darker than most expect due to the honey browning)

If you use honey (as I did in the photo) the pancakes will brown more. Also, the recipe above makes a loose batter; add more flour if you like a thicker pancake mix.

This recipe is a sneaky way to introduce whole-wheat berries into your diet. In a true emergency adjusting to a new diet would cause problems with your body's digestive system. If you do not have an emergency you can adapt this by using your coffee can grinder (or grain mill) to first grind the wheat, and then add the ingredients. But realize that the reason this tastes so much better than normal pancakes is that once the wheat is ground it starts to oxidize and lose flavor.

Week 20 Shopping List

To Buy:

❏ Camping or utility knife
❏ Work gloves
❏ Safety goggles
❏ Disposable dust masks
❏ 2 blank DVDs or flash drives
❏ An extra battery for motorized wheelchair or scooter, if needed

To Do:

❏ Use a video camera to tape the contents of your home for insurance purposes.
❏ Make a copy of the video and send to an out-of-town friend or family member.
❏ Find out about your workplace disaster plan.

Project 20:
How to Start a Fire with a Battery

Being a DIY prepper involves learning multiple disciplines, and although I believe living off the land in a wilderness setting is an unrealistic TEOTWAWKI (The End Of The World As We Know It) plan, I still think everyone should have basic wilderness survival skills. One outdoor skill everyone should possess is the ability to make fire.

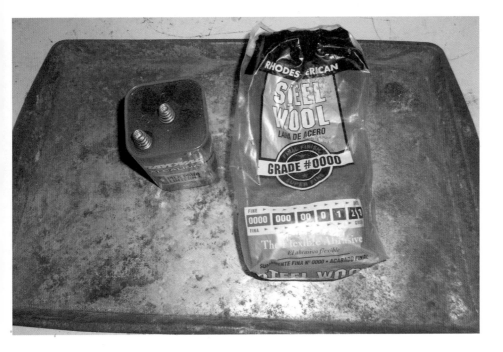

This is one skill in which redundancy is especially useful. Today's project involves using steel wool and a battery to light a fire. Once the basics are understood this process is repeatable with almost an unlimited variety of batteries. Theoretically, it can even be done using a remote control.

All you need to do is take a piece of fine steel wool—the finer the better (I use 0000 grade)—pull it apart a little to separate a few threads. To light it, take

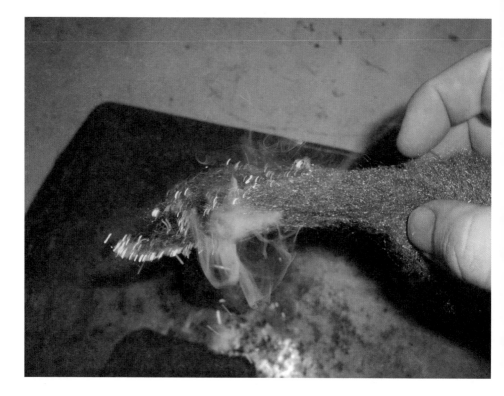

the steel wool threads and short-circuit a battery by connecting the wool to both battery terminals. Be careful, because the steel will immediately turn red hot. Blow on it a little and it will burst into flame. You can make it even more effective by mixing in a little dryer lint.

Once you have lit a fire with a lantern battery or a 9-volt battery and seen how easy it is, you can take the back off a flashlight, turn it on and use the battery and the metal flashlight case to do the same thing. Once you understand the science behind it, you can readily adapt it to other types of batteries. I have even repeated this process using cell phone batteries.

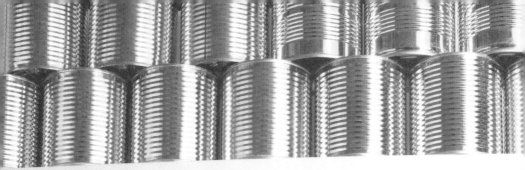

Week 21 Shopping List

At Week 21 we are finally done with our incremental shopping list. At this point you will have completed many activities that help better prepare your family, as well as have a fully stocked 72-hour kit. I urge you not to stop here but to continue to plan and prepare your family.

Congratulations on your accomplishment.

Project 21: Sumac Lemonade

This project is another "wilderness survival" project. We are going to take staghorn sumac and make a refreshing drink often called "sumac-ade." Sumacs grow throughout the world, with staghorn sumac (*Rhus hirta* or *Rhus glabra*) being the most common type.

Although we don't use it as a spice here in North America, sumac "stags" are used as a traditional spice in many cultures in the Middle East. If you dry and

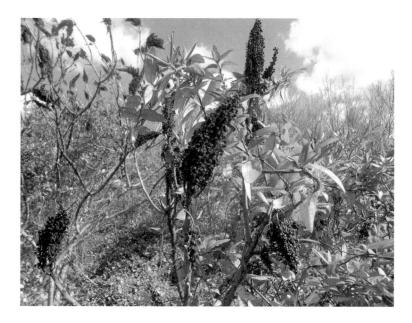

grind staghorn sumac you will find it has a tangy flavor that is often used with grilled meats and fish.

Though one should not eat wild food without first consulting a pictorial guide or an expert, it is very easy to distinguish staghorn sumac from poison sumac. The color of the berries is the biggest distinguisher.

Poison sumac has large white berries and only grows in wet areas—it is pretty rare.

Staghorn sumac has small red berries and is found all along country (and not so country) roads. I would bet that unless you live in a huge metropolis, you have seen sumac growing along the road.

Besides being a very cheap drink that tastes a lot like pink lemonade at a *fraction* of the cost, it has some health benefits, too. It is a good source of ascorbic acid—so preppers can use it to prevent scurvy. This alone makes it a worthwhile bit of information to have. It also has malic acid, calcium malate, dihydrofisetin, fisetin, iodine, gallic acid, tannic acid, selenium, and tartaric acid.

It has long been used as a folk medicine and has been the subject of research in modern medicine.

As far as a recipe—it's pretty much all to taste and pretty simple.

Ingredients:

- Sumac berries
- Water
- Sugar (to taste)

Preparation

- Pick the sumac around August in order to make sure it is ripe.
- Don't pick the sumac cones after rain since the flavor comes from the sap on the outside of the berries.

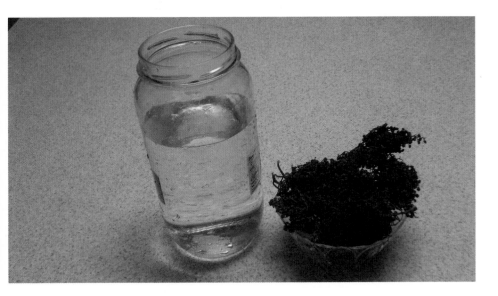

- Remove as many leaves and twigs as possible. The more stems, the more tannic acid you will get.
- Place the sumac berries in a container filled with fresh cold water. You'll want about 1 cup of water for each cone. Warm water will make your drink bitter.
- Crush the berries with your hands.
- Let rest for about 30–60 minutes depending on how strong of a flavor you want.
- Strain using cheesecloth and sweeten to your liking. Serve cold with ice.

Personally, while I have to have sugar in my tea, I don't feel that sumac-ade needs sweeteners.

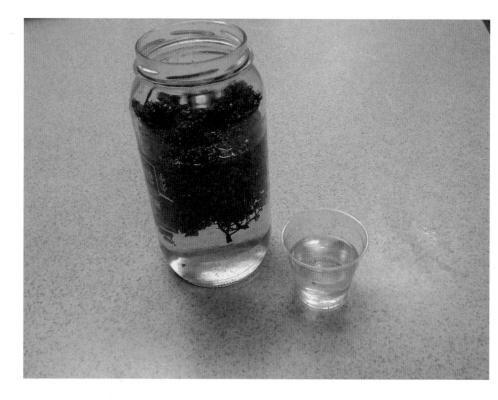

Project 22: Raised Bed Garden

So far I have not proven my skills as a grower of plants. This is something I am working diligently to change. In a catastrophic disaster or economic collapse the ability to produce food is something that will be necessary for survival. Besides

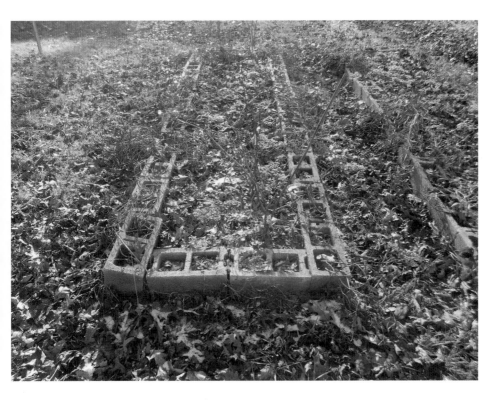

that, growing your own food has additional benefits for healthier living, a more economic lifestyle, and the pleasure that comes from producing it.

As I have spent several thousands of dollars in gardening plans for little produce I am not so sure about gardening being cheaper, but I still hold out hope.

My front yard is the sunniest part of my yard, and really the only area I have to grow food. But since my yard is mostly clay and I did not want to go through the process of amending the soil I decided to make a raised bed.

New cinderblocks cost $1.07 each at the time I made the beds. I used 102 of them.

My intent was to keep the inner dimensions 10x2 so I could utilize square foot gardening techniques.

I made each row 11 blocks long with two blocks separating each row, which made the outer dimension 11x3 and the inner 10x2. I also decided to fill in the centers of the blocks to give me additional growing space. In an area of frost upheaval, you might want to put the blocks on their sides. You will lose growing space, but they won't fill with water and crack.

My calculations tell me the cubic feet of topsoil needed for the beds would be near 4 cubic yards. I added extra for the block centers and ordered 6 yards to ensure I had some left over to use for other projects.

I find that building the beds is much easier (and more fun) then filling them with dirt. It took me about 5 wheelbarrow loads of dirt to fill each bed, and after the beds were full I came back and added another couple loads to the top to smooth the bed level and fill the side holes.

I hope to be able to brag on my produce this year. But just let me warn you, buying a paint can of "survival seeds" is a *bad* idea—if you ever have to open the can you're going to use *a lot* of energy breaking your yard up for planting— you probably won't have access to the materials needed to build a garden, and you may not have the skills to keep the plants alive (or in my case, keep from killing them).

It is much better to learn this skill now. It is not something you learn from a book without putting in the work.

Project 23:
Survival Squirrel Snare

Trapping gives much more meat per unit of energy expended than hunting does. Using snares is a passive activity; you can set several traps in multiple locations and check them once a day, leaving you free to do other useful work while still gathering food. Hunting requires active attention; you cannot stalk a deer while tending a signal fire.

Snares are also relatively lightweight, cheap, and easy to pack.

Today's project shows how to make and use a small game snare using bailing wire or 20-gauge galvanized steel wire.

A roll of this wire is about $5, makes several dozen snares, is relatively lightweight and compact, and can be used for other survival uses.

Procedure:

• Cut a length of wire approximately 18 inches long (length depends on how you are going to attach it).
• Make a small loop at one end of the wire.
• Run the wire back over itself and through the small twisted loop you made. This makes a larger loop "lasso." The wire should run freely through the

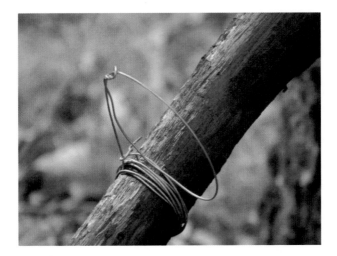

small twisted loop you made at the end of the wire. The loop this forms should be approximately the diameter of a Coke can.

- With the small twisted loop at approximately the "10 o'clock" position, run the free end of your wire snare down and attach it to your squirrel run.
- The squirrel run is a straight stick relatively free of limbs and 6–10 feet long. It should be about the same thickness as a man's wrist. This branch has one end resting on the ground and the other resting on the trunk of a tree. It should intersect the ground at an approximate 45-degree angle.

If possible, you want to pick a tree that has a squirrel nest in it, or is an oak tree – that way squirrels will be naturally drawn to it.

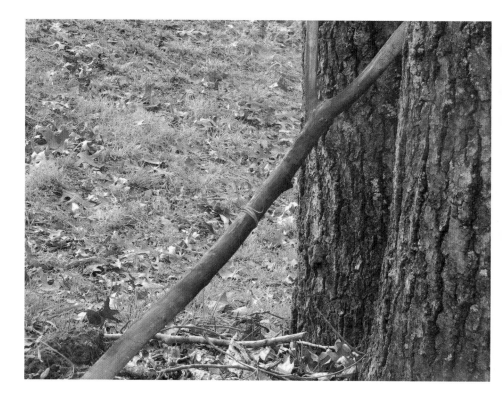

The idea is that a squirrel will choose to run up the stick to get to the tree trunk, as that is easier for it to get on the tree than jumping the 90 degree angle to move from ground to trunk.

If a squirrel runs up the pole it will have to move through the snare. It won't mind as it looks flexible and the squirrel can see through it. As it enters the snare, its head goes in, but its body cannot. The snare tightens around it as it runs it hits the end of the wire and falls off the branch in its struggle.

If the wire is placed appropriately, it will hang itself and will not be able to climb back up.

You can place multiple snares on a single run; just make sure they are all high enough that a snared squirrel will hang free and not touch the ground, and that there is enough space that they cannot touch each other.

Before doing this, you need to look at the game laws in your area. In my state of Tennessee, this is illegal, and not something I would do as long as I can go to the grocery for food. But in the event nothing else was available and I would starve otherwise, there are many squirrels in my subdivision (or nearby parks) and they could mean the difference between going hungry or not.

Project 24:
How to Eat Acorns

Acorns have been tested and found to be one of the best foods for effectively controlling blood sugar levels. They have low sugar content, but leave a sweetish aftertaste, making them very good in stews, as well as in breads of all types.

The only two problems I have with eating acorns are that I am too lazy to pick them up quickly enough to prevent worms from ruining them, and that the tannins give them a bitter taste. Luckily there are solutions to both problems, and this project will teach you them.

This year I decided to harvest acorns from the oak trees in my front yard. Being lazy, I spread out a large tarp and weighted it down with rocks. Every afternoon (or so) from September to early November I would take a quick look and scoop up any acorns I saw on the tarp. If the acorns were soft feeling or looked like they were compromised, I tossed them down the hill; the good ones went inside with me to collect in a place where they would not be subject to rot or worms.

Once I got enough acorns to make the process worthwhile I processed them to remove the tannins. Tannic acid makes the acorns bitter, but different oak trees have differing amounts of tannins in the acorns. Depending on the oak tree and your taste buds, it may be possible to eat the acorns without any processing.

Unfortunately, oaks with that low of a tannin level are rare (Native Americans fought wars over them). They are also normally found on the West Coast. Beware that eating acorns without removing the tannins will make your mouth feel like cotton, can cause constipation, and, with large amounts, can even cause kidney damage. Luckily, to process your acorns all you really need is water.

Native Americans basically threw their acorns in baskets and left them in swiftly running streams until the tannins were leeched out. For us modern folks, there are faster ways.

First thing to do is dry them out so that they don't mold. You can lay them out on a sheet or tarp, single layer deep, and let the sun cook them. Personally, I would rather throw them in the dehydrator for a couple hours, or put them on a cookie sheet in the oven at its lowest temperature (about 175 degrees Fahrenheit) for about an hour.

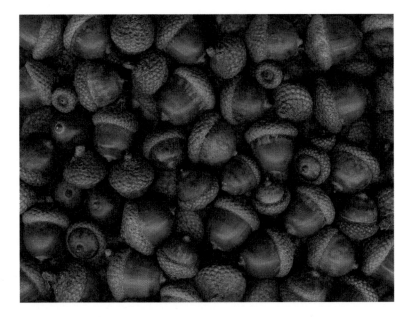

Next, peel the acorn; it's simple to crack the shell with a nutcracker or slip joint pliers, peel off the thin skin, and throw the good acorns in a bucket. If the acorn has a black hole it is evidence of worm infestation—throw those out.

Next, get your food grinder and make a course meal. Put the meal in a pot and cover with boiling water. After an hour the water should be brown to black. You can throw this out; however, I have heard of using the tannin water

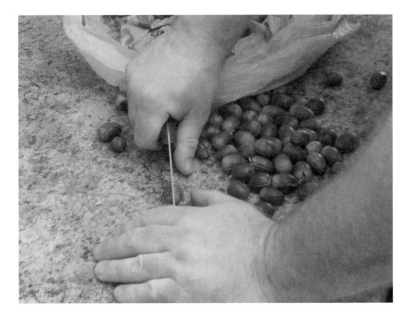

to tan animal hides. Taste the meal: if it tastes sweet, it's done; if it's like eating a green persimmon, repeat the boiling water soak. Do this as many times as necessary.

Once you are happy with the meal, lay it out to dry. A good way to start this process is to dump the wet meal in a sheet or doubled sheet of cheesecloth, gather the ends like a jelly bag, and press the water out. Next, put it in the oven at its lowest setting or in a dehydrator. Be careful with this process, as if you let the meal sit around wet it will mold.

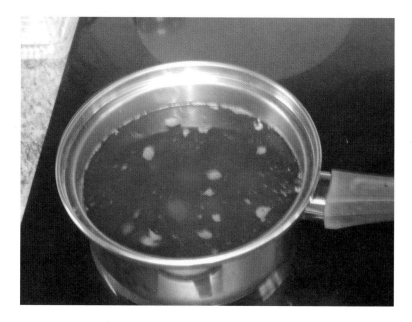

In an airtight jar the coarsely ground chunks will last a while in the freezer. Grind it to flour as you need it, because the acorn oil will go rancid about as fast as whole grains will. Either way, course or fine, it will start go rancid in a couple weeks if stored at room temperature.

You can use acorn meal in many of the same ways as wheat flour. I have seen recipes online for acorn pasta, pancakes, and various breads.

Project 25: Sprouting Wheat and Beans

We all know that nothing is free, especially food storage. Finding foods that are cost effective and long storing generally means you have less of the two vs—variety and vitamins. Sprouting is a way to add both. I used to associate sprouts with homeopathic medicine practitioners, vegans, and yuppie soccer moms, but once I got over my initial prejudice I learned that it's simple and cheap to add sprouts to my food toolbox.

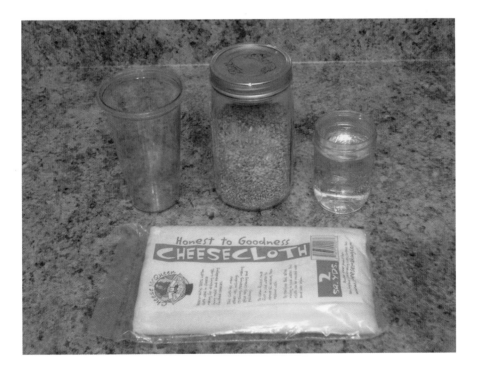

Studies show that sprouts have 3 to 5 times the vitamin content of the seed they sprouted from. And as for vitamins, sprouts have over 30 times the vitamin

C content of the original seed. Wheat grain sprouts have a lot of vitamins and also have a good amount of protein and enzymes. The great thing about wheat is that due to the enzyme actions in the seed as it sprouts, your body is able to use the nutrients inside.

There are all sorts of recipes online for sprouts, and I would suggest you try a couple now and see how easy it is to incorporate sprouts into your everyday food. Personally, I like adding them to my salad, but my favorite way of using them is feeding them to my chickens and eating the eggs they produce. . . .

How to Use Sprouted Wheat:
- Add either chopped or whole to homemade bread
- Add to oatmeal or other whole grain cereal
- Stir into cooked rice
- Add to rice pilaf
- Knead into pizza dough
- Chop and add to cookies
- Add to muffins, pancakes, and waffles (like our whole wheat pancakes)
- Add to casseroles, stuffed peppers, meatloaf, meatballs, pasta sauce, and mushroom sauces
- Add to sandwiches
- Sprinkle on yogurt
- Sprinkle in salads
- In stir fry

Equipment:
- Wide-mouthed jar (or something similar)
- Nylon net or cheesecloth and rubber band (to cover the jar and keep the cover in place)

Ingredients:
- ½ cup wheat berries
- Water

Procedure:
- Rinse ½ cup of wheat berries.
- Put the wheat berries in a wide-mouth quart jar.

Don't put too many berries in the jar—no more than ½ cup per wide-mouth jar.

- Add 2 cups of room temperature water.
- Place nylon net or cheesecloth over the jar opening.

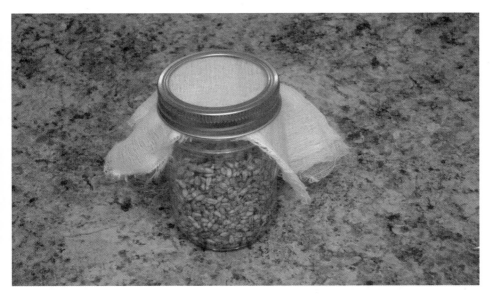

- Use a heavy rubber band or the metal jar ring to hold the nylon or cheesecloth in place.
- Soak 12 hours, then drain.
- Thoroughly drain the water—shake a bit to remove most of the water.
- Keep the jar out of direct sunlight.
- It needs the air, so keep cheesecloth as a lid.
- Each morning and night rinse the wheat berries with room temperature water, drain again. Taste after each soaking, Some keep the liquid drained off and drink it; I have done this, but I don't like the taste—even if I did feel a burst of energy after drinking it.
- 36 to 48 hours after the first soaking, voila! You have germinated wheat, and if you continue the process for a day or two more you will have sprouted wheat.

Storing Wheat Sprouts:

Replace the nylon net or cheesecloth with plastic wrap or the metal jar lid to help keep it moist but not wet. Store in cool place for no more than 5 days.

Project 26:
Pressure Canner Cooking

In any disaster situation, energy is a premium. If you are cooking over a fire, every second of heat is paid for several times over with work finding, carrying, chopping, and stacking firewood. If you are using a petroleum-based fuel you have to rely on your supply, which is something you may not be able to replace easily. Therefore, anything you can do to cook your food faster is something to consider. Besides energy costs, time saved cooking is time gained to take care of other things (which is useful outside of a disaster too).

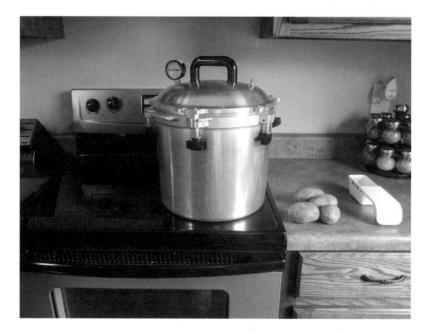

Today's project is one such time-saving method of cooking. For simplicity's sake we are going to use potatoes in our project—but as you can see from the chart below, this method of cooking works with all manners of foods.

Cooking Times Chart

Obviously many factors will influence your cooking times. Use this information as a guideline, but the actual cooking times may vary depending on your pressure cooker, heat source, and the quality and/or quantity of the food.

All times are for 15 psi pressure using a cooking rack.

For most vegetables, the cold water release method is recommended for tender-crisp results, and the quick release will produced a more "cooked" result. Dense vegetables like whole potatoes, yams, or winter squash can benefit from the natural release. For instructions on the release method, please look at the instructions at the end of the chart.

Vegetables	Cooking Time (Minutes)	Liquid (Cups)	Release
Artichoke, hearts	2 to 3	½	Cold water
Asparagus, thin whole	1 to 1½	½	Cold water
Beans, green or wax	2 to 3	½	Natural release
Beets, small whole	12	½	Natural release
Broccoli, florets	2 to 3	½	Cold water
Broccoli stalks, ¼-inch slices	3 to 4	½	Cold water
Brussels sprouts, small	3	½	Cold water
Cabbage, any variety—quartered	3 to 4	½	Cold water
Carrots, whole	3 to 5	½	Natural release
Carrots, 1-inch chunks	4	½	Cold water
Cauliflower, whole	6	½	Cold water
Celery, 1-inch slices	3	½	Cold water
Corn, kernels	1	½	Cold water
Corn on the cob	4	½	Cold water
Eggplant, sliced ⅛- to ¼-inch slices	2 to 3	½	Cold water
Endive, thickly cut	1 to 2	½	Cold water
Escarole, coarsely chopped	1 to 2	½	Cold water

Vegetables	Cooking Time (Minutes)	Liquid (Cups)	Release
Greens, Beet, coarsely chopped	1 to 4	½	Cold water
Greens, Collard coarsely chopped	5	½	Cold water
Greens, Kale, coarsely chopped	1 to 2	½	Cold water
Greens, Kohlrabi, cut	3 to 4	½	Cold water
Greens, Mustard, cut in pieces	3 to 4	½	Cold water
Greens, Swiss chard, coarsely chopped	2	½	Cold water
Greens, Turnip greens, coarsely chopped	4	½	Cold water
Leeks, whole, large (white part only)	3 to 4	½	Cold water
Mixed vegetables	2	½	Cold water
Okra, small pods	2 to 3	½	Cold water
Onions, whole	7 to 9	½	Cold water
Onions, quartered	3	½	Cold water
Parsnips, 1-inch chunks	4	½	Cold water
Parsnips, ¼-inch cubes	2	½	Cold water
Peas, shelled	1	½	Cold water
Pepper, whole, sweet or bell	3	½	Cold water
Potatoes, new or small (2-inch diameter), whole	8	½	Natural release
Potatoes, red, whole	10	½	Natural release
Potatoes, red, halved	6	½	Natural release
Potatoes, red, cubed	4	½	Cold water
Potatoes, large baking-size, whole	25	1	Natural release
Pumpkin, 2-inch chunks	3 to 4	½	Cold water
Rutabagas, 1-inch chunks, peeled	4	½	Cold water

Vegetables	Cooking Time (Minutes)	Liquid (Cups)	Release
Rutabagas, 2-inch cuts, peeled	6 to 8	½	Natural release
Spinach, coarsely chopped	1	½	Cold water
Spinach, whole leaves	0	½	Cold water
Squash, Acorn, halved	8	½	Cold water
Squash, Banana, cubed	3 to 4	½	Cold water
Squash, Butternut, 1-inch chunks	4	½	Cold water
Squash, Butternut, halves	6	½	Cold water
Squash, Chayote or Merliton, halved	5	½	Cold water
Squash, Spaghetti, 2 lbs. whole or halves	9	½	Cold water
Squash, Summer or Yellow, ½ inch slices	0	½	Cold water
Squash, Zucchini, 1½-inch slices	2 to 3	½	Cold water
Tomatoes, quartered	2	½	Cold water
Tomatoes, whole	3	½	Cold water
Turnips, small, quartered	8	½	Cold water
Turnips, ½-inch chunks	5	½	Cold water
Yams, ½-inch slices	6	½	Cold water

Cold Water Release Method

This is the fastest method, used to immediately stop the cooking process by lowering the heat *and* the temperature. If an immediate release of pressure *and* temperature is desired, the pot is carried to the sink and cold water is run over the lid (but not the valve).

Always position the cooker in the sink so that it is tilted at a slight angle. Let the cold stream of water run over top of the lid, but not directly over the vent pipe or valve, letting it run down the side of the cooker to cool it quickly.

If your faucet is too short to allow water to run over the top of the cooker, use the sprayer attachment if available; otherwise, partially fill with sink with cold water before setting the cooker in it.

This method is mainly used for food with very short cooking times, or where it is essential to stop the cooking process as fast as possible. Use this method for serving fresh, tender-crisp vegetables, or delicate seafood. Owners of electric pressure cookers do not have the cold water option, and that limits some of the foods and recipes they can cook.

Precautions for the Cold Water Release Method

Never run water directly over the pressure release vent or valve when using the cold water release method. Direct the water to the outer edge of the lid so that it runs down the side of the pot. A variation on this method is to fill the sink with several inches of cold water and then sit the pressure cooker in the cold water bath. (When the pressure cooker is removed from heat the air molecules inside the pot begin to cool and contract, and if the vent opening is blocked by the stream of water, then no air molecules can get inside to replace the volume. The air inside the cooker rapidly contracts as it cools so there is less air pressure inside the pot than outside. This creates a very powerful vacuum that can actually cause the lid (or the weakest area of the metal) to collapse as the vacuum sucks it down inside the pot).

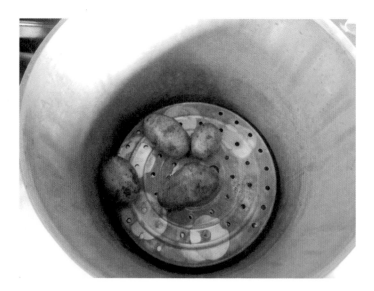

Natural Release Method

This is the slowest method to gradually drop the pressure and the temperature to finish the cooking process. (This is the only method to use when you are canning.)

In this method you remove the pot from the heat source to allow the pressure to subside naturally. If you are cooking beans, potatoes, or other foods that have skins that you wish to remain intact, this is the preferred method.

Use this release method for foods that increase in volume, froth, or foam, or those that are mostly liquids, like soup or broth. Most meats and other long-cooking recipes are finished this way to complete the cooking process.

If you own an electric model, keep in mind that the heating element will retain heat and that will prolong the cool down period-which may result in foods that are overcooked.

Precautions for the Natural Method

The food inside the cooker continues to cook throughout this slow cool down process. This method is commonly used for finishing large cuts of meat, foods that foam froth or expand during cooking, and foods that are mostly liquid, such as stock or broth. The natural release method should not be used for delicate vegetables or fish, or any food or recipe with very short cooking times.

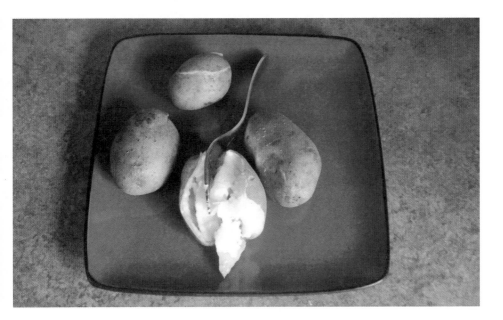

Project 27: Pressure Canning Beans

Having the ability to pressure can is a vital skill: It allows you to buy (or produce) food in bulk and store it for several years without having to use a freezer. Canned food can be eaten directly from the can, and in the case of dry beans, the final product can be of a better quality than the normal cooking methods.

Pressure-cooking requires attention to detail and adherence to reliable recipes. When done correctly pressure canning is safe, as the internal temperatures become high enough to kill any bacteria that are naturally present in the food. It is also much more flexible than water-bath canning because it allows for canning low acid foods like meat and beans.

If you are new to canning, here are a few caveats:

• You need to get dial-based canners calibrated/checked each year. Normally the county agriculture service will do this for free.
• If you have a choice, buy a canner that uses a top and bottom that are machined for an airtight fit, rather than one that relies on a gasket. Gaskets break, and sometimes replacements are hard to find.
• Use scientifically tested recipes. Just because someone's grandma never succumbed to botulism poisoning does not mean that her recipe kills botulism spores.
• You need to devote time to the canning process so you can watch the dial on the canner. If it rises too high it can rupture; if it drops below the pressures designated in the recipe you have to bring it back up to the correct pressure and restart your timer.
• A higher pressure and a longer time may ensure that any organisms present in the food are killed, but it also has a negative effect on taste and texture. Only use the times and pressures listed in the recipes.

Why can dried beans? I will give you a couple reasons. The first is that it gives you storage options. I don't like putting all my eggs in one basket, and by canning beans and storing them dry I have two separate ways of getting at the same foodstuff. The next reason is that by canning them ahead of time I cut down on prep time. It takes hours of cooking to soften dried beans, but it only takes 90 minutes to pressure can beans, and then they are ready to eat right from the jar, or reheated with a minimum of fuel resources.

Pressure canned beans are almost always soft and tender, while it can be hard to get dried beans soft enough for my taste, especially if they have been in long-term storage. Lastly, in a disaster situation, I may not have the time to tend to a pot of beans cooking all day, nor the refrigeration to keep the leftovers from spoiling. With a can of beans, it's a serving per can, with no leftovers, and very little time spent reheating them.

Because dried beans are a low-acid food they require processing in a pressure canner. Before attempting to can dried beans, or any low-acid food, make sure you are familiar with the steam-pressure canning process as well as the specific recommendations for your particular pressure canner. Some, but not all, pressure cookers can be used for pressure canning. Before using a pressure cooker for pressure canning purposes, make sure it is suitable for such use.

In the recipe below I specify pinto beans; however, other dried beans can also be canned with this method.

Depending on the desired use, other seasonings can be added, and both the salt and the seasoning are optional ingredients and can be left out if desired.

If you are concerned about flatulence, a little lemon juice or citric acid in the soak will help break up the enzymes that cause the problem.

A 1-pound package of dried beans will produce around 5 pints of canned beans.

Recipe

• Wash beans and remove any stones or dirt clods.
• Place beans in a pot and cover with cold water by 2 inches.
• Let beans stand in a cool place for 12 hours.

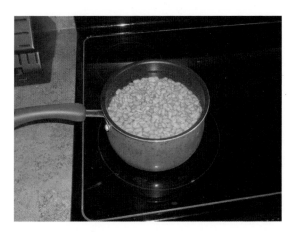

- Drain beans and rinse with fresh water.
- Return beans to pot and add water to cover by 2 inches.
- Bring beans to a boil over medium heat and continue boiling for 30 minutes.
- Pack hot beans into hot canning jars, leaving 1-inch headspace.

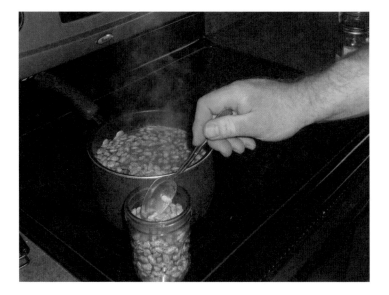

- Add ½ teaspoon salt to each pint or 1 teaspoon to each quart.

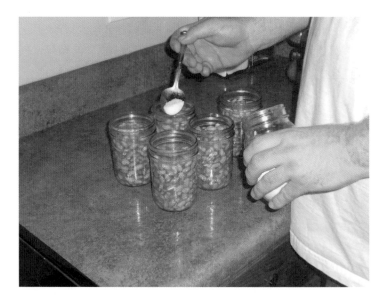

- Ladle hot cooking liquid over beans, leaving 1-inch headspace.
- Remove bubbles and wipe jar rim to remove any broth. Adjust two-piece caps.

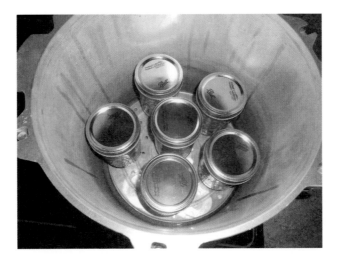

- Process pints 75 minutes, quarts 90 minutes, in a steam-pressure canner at 10 pounds pressure.

Remember that processing times depend on your elevation, and that you must process for the required time to kill any bacterial spores. Always follow a recipe approved by the USDA or canner manufacturer.

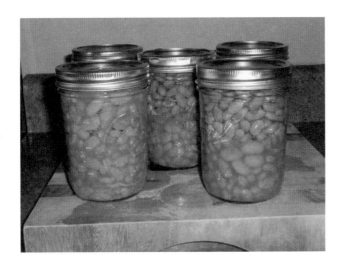

Project 28: Making a Top Bar Beehive

When I decided on beekeeping I wanted to build my own hive, and I had decided on building a Kenyan hive, or a Top Bar Hive (TBH). This type of hive was designed by missionaries and aide workers in Kenya because of the simplicity of design. It is popular here because it is a much more natural way of beekeeping, and the thought is that if the bees can build their hive how they want to, then they will naturally do what is needed to prevent beetles and mites.

You get less honey with a top bar hive than with a traditional hive because the bees don't have the benefit of foundation, and because each time you gather honey you have to destroy the comb, so they have to make more comb, which takes up many more pounds of honey. (That's not a problem for me, as I *want* the wax—I bought several candle molds, and beeswax makes great bullet lube for reloading.) TBH comb also has to be handled more gently, as there is no frame to hold it in place, so if you are not careful it will break off and fall—ruining the honey, and royally ticking off the bees.

Making a hive is pretty simple: all you need is a box, a way to keep the box off the ground, top bars, and a cover to keep rain out of the hive. As you build your box, consider building it with a 30-degree angle instead of a 90 degree, because the bees don't like attaching comb at angles, so you won't get as much comb being stuck to the sides of the hive, and because it is easier to lift the comb out of an inverted triangle without hitting the sides of the hive.

As you cut your top bars, ensure that they fit flush against the top of the hive, so that bees cannot get up and over the bars and glue them to the roof. Also, the bars do not have to hold a lot of weight, so make them relatively thin: the thicker they are, the more likely you are to smash bees as you move the bars around.

Parts:

Use untreated lumber (treated or painted lumber will either kill your bees or make them leave).

• Two ¾-inch boards, 12 inches wide and cut 15 inches long
• Two ¾-inch boards, 12 inches wide and cut 36 inches long
• Thirty ¾-inch boards, ripped 1⅜ inches wide and 17 inches long
• Marine-grade plywood
• Large brick
• Hardware cloth
• Wood screws
• Beeswax

Instructions:

• Measure and mark 2 ½ inches from each bottom corner on the long side of the 2 12x15 inch boards.
• Draw a line from the top right corner to the right most bottom mark, and then draw a line from the top left corner to the left bottom mark.
• Saw along both lines, and repeat the process on the other board. This creates the end pieces and will measure 15 inches across the top and 10 inches along the bottom.
• Drill several ¾ inch holes in one of the end pieces. These holes are the hive entrance holes and should be located at the center of the end board from the middle point down.

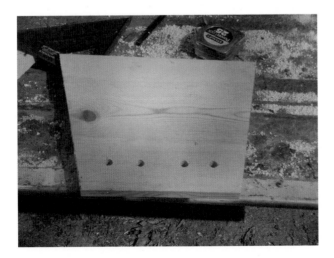

- Using wood screws, attach the 36-inch boards to each side of the end pieces to form a box.

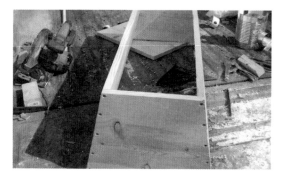

- Staple a sheet of hardware cloth to the bottom of the box. This helps with mites and temperature regulation. Depending on your climate, you may need to set the hive on a board (or otherwise enclose the bottom) in the winter to keep the hive warm.

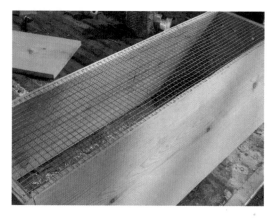

- Rip the bars. Cut 30 boards that are ¾ inch by 1 ⅜ inches by 17 inches. Set two bars aside, then mark a line down the center of each board, leaving 2 inches at each end. The unmarked bars are empty spacer bars for each end of the hive.
- Cut a groove along those lines. You could use a circular saw set for a shallow cut, or a carving tool to create the grooves that are at least ⅛ inch deep.
- Pour melted beeswax into the grooves. This creates a base for the bees to start building their own wax combs. Leaving the edges clean prevents the bees from attaching the comb to the walls of the hive.

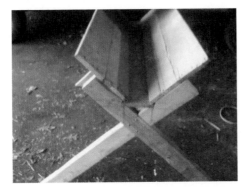

- Place a clean bar at each end of the hive, then lay the waxed bars across the top of the box, waxed side down, until the top is covered.
- You can paint or otherwise weatherproof the outside of the hive, but nothing should be painted on the top bars or inside the hive.
- Cut a section of marine plywood, roofing material, or other waterproof medium to lay on the hive to keep out weather. Weight this down with a large brick
- Set the hive in a level sunny area, at least a foot above the ground. (I set several on a 2x4 frame balanced on cinder blocks.)

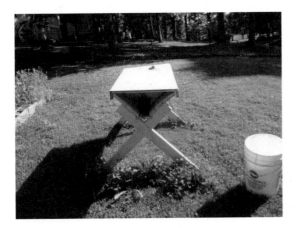

Depending on state law, you will probably have to register your hives, but the only things you need to get started are a package of bees, a smoker, and a veil.

This is the cheapest way to start beekeeping, and will quickly help you decide if you want to expand your hobby.

Beekeeping is not hard, and once you start having your own honey, you will be *very* popular with your neighbors.

Project 29:
Beginning Cheese Making

Cheese making may be a project that some skip over, or it may ignite into a full-fledged hobby. Traditionally cheese making was a way to store milk. It is much simpler than I expected, and was the project that broke the confidence barrier. Once I made my own cheese and said "I can do this," I was much more willing to try more complex projects.

Normally most cheese makers use liquid milk, either store bought or from a farm, but once you get the basics down you can adapt. In a later project you learn how to make cheese from the powdered milk that most preppers store but don't really know what to do with.

Personally, I could live without electricity more easily than I could without cheese.

Homemade Mozzarella

If you want to try cheese making at home, I highly recommend Ricki Carroll's book *Home Cheese Making: Recipes for 75 Delicious Cheeses*. I own it and think the recipes are well thought out to be as simple as possible.

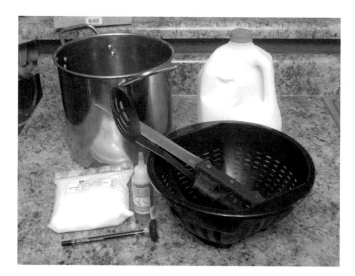

This is a simple recipe and pretty easy to make as long as you follow the recipe step by step. My only disaster was when I was trying to tape the procedure and spent too much time talking and not enough doing.

Equipment:

- 1 gallon pot—stainless steel or enameled
- Thermometer
- Colander
- Slotted spoon
- Long knife
- Microwavable bowl

Ingredients:

- 1 gallon milk
- 1 ½ teaspoon citric acid dissolved in 1 cup chlorine-free water
- ¼ rennet dissolved in ¼ cup chlorine-free water
- 1 tablespoon of cheese salt and/or herbs (optional—but I found it bland without salt)

Directions:

- Pour milk into pot and vigorously stir ion citric acid.

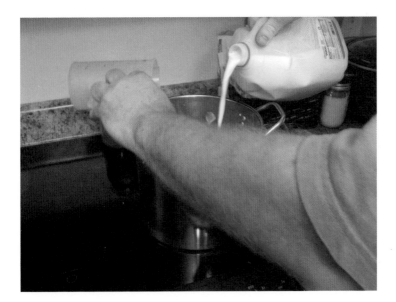

- Heat to 90 degrees Fahrenheit while stirring.
- Remove from heat and stir in the rennet solution with a dashing motion (up and down like making butter in an old-fashioned dasher) for about 30 seconds.

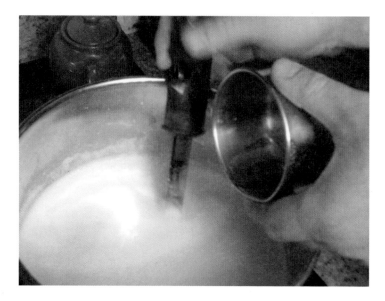

- Cover pot and let sit for 5 minutes.
- If the curd looks like a white Jell-O with a clear separation of the curd and the whey, cut the curd into ½-inch "blocks."

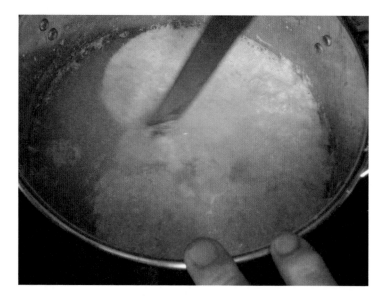

- Heat the curds to 105 degrees Fahrenheit while gently stirring.
- Take off burner and stir for another 2–5 minutes (longer time = firmer finished cheese).
- Pour off floating whey (save it for bread making).
- Ladle curds into large microwavable bowl and drain as much whey as possible without pressing curds too hard (you can press down a little, but don't mash it flat).

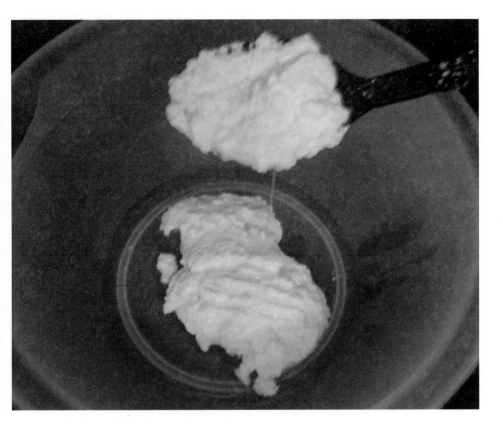

- Microwave bowl for 1 minute.
- Alternatively, instead of microwaving cheese, just dunk it in hot water repeatedly. The idea is to keep the cheese hot while you work it.
- Remove and drain as you gently fold curds into a single piece. (Add salt now if desired.)
- Microwave for another 30 seconds. Drain and stretch.
- Cheese must be 135 degrees Fahrenheit to stretch—if it is not hot enough, microwave for another 30 seconds.

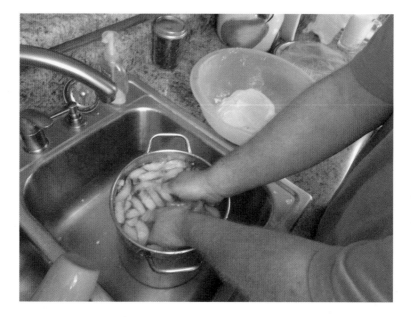

- I used latex gloves to help with heat, as well as having an ice bath nearby to dip my hands in occasionally.
- Keep stretching cheese like taffy—the more you heat and stretch, the firmer it will be.
- When finished stretching submerge it in ice water to set the cheese.

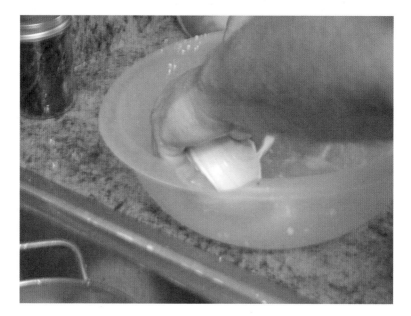

Submerging the cheese is critical for texture and to prevent it from being grainy.

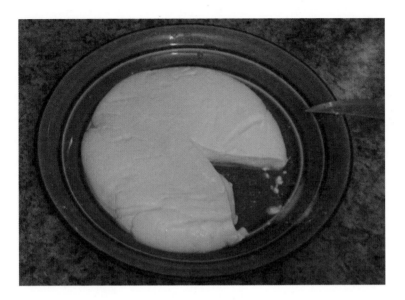

Alternatives to Cheesecloth

Cheesecloth is cotton—so any undyed cotton of the proper weave would probably work. You could also try nylon as a substitute.

• Cheesecloth is generally 60 threads per square inch
• Butter Muslin is generally 90 threads per inch

I have tried several types of cloth in making cheese:

• Nylon tulle mesh costs me about $1.97 per yard
• Unbleached cotton muslin costs me about $1.50 a yard
• Bleached cotton costs me about $0.97 a yard

The muslin and cotton worked well with the strained yogurt. The tulle worked great for large curd cheese or straining honey.

What worked the best was a $4.50 beer wort straining bag that I bought at the brewing supply store.

You need to understand what you want to accomplish and then be flexible enough mentally that you can adapt when you cannot find something that is labeled exactly how you expect.

Project 30:
Making Soft Curd Cheese from Powdered Milk

This project is pretty easy—it's basically the same as making ricotta cheese.

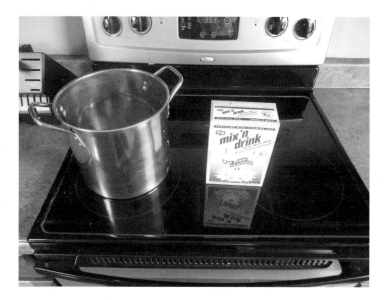

If this interests you, then I recommend you buy the book *Cooking with Home Storage* by Peggy Layton and Vicki Tate, which has many recipes like this, including a similar recipe for making "mock mozzarella" in a similar method that adds hanging the curds in a cheesecloth. I have this book and many others by Mrs. Tate, and believe they are well worth the money.

As with most things, fat makes everything taste better, so if you have whole milk powder, your cheese will have a richer taste. Unfortunately, almost all milk stored long term is the nonfat kind, as the milk fats cause the powdered milk to go rancid very quickly. As a matter of fact, dry milk from your grocery is probably either already rancid or very close to its 6-month shelf life. This is one item that I recommend buying from specialty disaster prep stores. This way the product was packaged in #10 cans immediately after manufacture.

Equipment:

- Large stainless steel stock pot
- Long-handled stainless steel spoon
- Cheesecloth
- Colander

Ingredients:

- 3 cups powdered milk
- 6 cups water
- Vinegar

Instructions:

- Reconstitute your dried milk; you can either follow the directions on the milk package or combine 3 cups of powdered milk with 6 cups of cold water in a large stock pot. Stir until the milk is totally dissolved in the water.
- Heat the milk over medium low heat until it reaches 120 degrees Fahrenheit. You need a good cooking thermometer to make cheese, but if you don't have one yet, heat the milk until it is hot to the touch, but not scalding.
- Turn off the heat and add ¼ cup of vinegar to the milk.
- Stir and let the milk sit for 10 minutes.

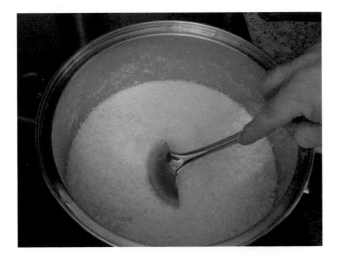

- You should see the curds separate from the whey; if not add an additional ¼ cup of vinegar and wait another 10 minutes.

There are also some neat recipes online (http://www.sciencebob.com/experiments/plasticmilk.php) for making a very primitive plastic using a very similar method. I find it to be a neat science demonstration for kids, but I find it to be too brittle for any real use.

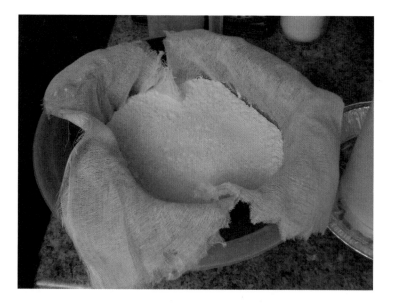

- Place a sheet of cheesecloth in a colander. Pour the curds into the cheesecloth.
- If desired, set the colander over a large bowl and collect the whey.
- Rinse the cheese curds under cold running water and let drain. Transfer to a covered container and store in the refrigerator.

Whey is useful for replacing water in many recipes like:

- Baking
- Soups
- Soaking grains
- Smoothies and shakes
- Watering your garden
- I find that the dog really likes it (it has a lot of proteins).

Project 31:
DIY $20 Cheese Press

To me, preparedness is more about attitudes and skills than gear and gadgets. The way that I build those skills is to create a sustainable lifestyle that allows me the ability to learn new things and then practice them.

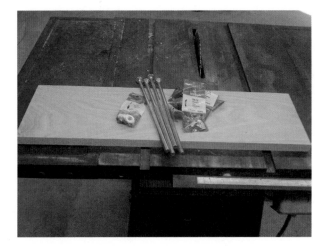

By now you have noticed several cheese projects. They were not selected because making homemade cheese is cheaper than store-bought cheese (it's generally not), or because I think you have to have cheese to survive "The End Of the World As We Know It" (even if it's a good way of storing milk without refrigerators).

I am taking the time to post about cheese making because it is a good do-it-yourself skill that is fun and easy, but allows the prepper to start moving and planning, while teaching skills such as patience and how to plan for the future (it takes 6 months or more to see the benefits of a hard cheddar).

Now that you have made a couple easy soft cheeses, some of the next projects will leverage that skill and confidence into making hard cheese, but you will need a new tool. This project is how to make a cheese press.

This cheese press is very simple and easy to make (around $10–$20), which is nice because more complex presses can cost hundreds of dollars.

Parts:

- Two food-grade hardwood boards, approximately 12–18 inches long, ½ to ¾ inch thick, and 6–8 inches wide. Normally a store such as Lowes or Home Depot will have this in the craft wood aisle, and will cut a longer board into sections for you.
- 4 carriage bolts, as long as you can find (must be longer than your cheese mold, both boards, washers and nuts, and around ½ inch in diameter). If you cannot find a long enough bolt, you can use threaded rod and twice as many nuts. Stainless works best.
- Wing nuts and washers for the bolts. Like the bolts, stainless is more expensive but safer for food. Galvanized will discolor over time as it contacts the cheese.
- Cheese mold
- Weights, in 1-pound increments to 20 pounds
- Aluminum pie plate

Instructions:

- Drill ½-inch holes at each corner of the boards. They need to line up with both boards and be far enough from the edge of the board so as not to split.

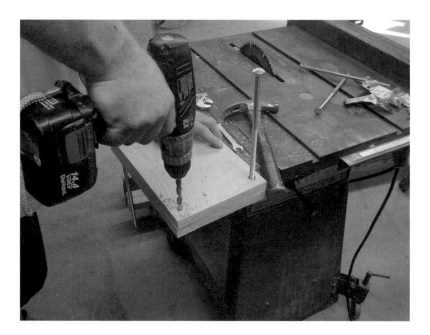

- Thread carriage bolt up through one board so that ends of bolts become the "feet" of the cheese press.
- Insert second board over bolts, and thread washers and wing nuts on to bolts.
- Lay aluminum plate over board and cut one side slightly to allow whey to drain away from cheese curd.

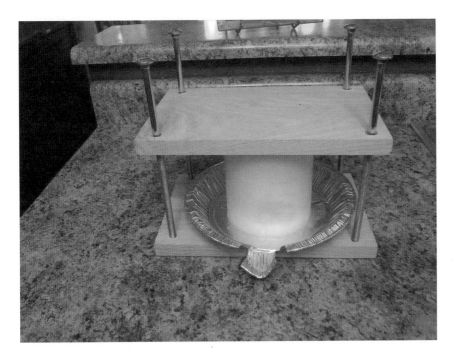

Use:

- To use press, fill cheese mold with cheesecloth-wrapped curds (as described in next project).
- Place mold and pie plate on bottom board, and cover with second board making a sandwich of board, plate, mold, and board.
- Lightly tighten wing nut. You are not using nuts to press out liquid whey but to keep everything together.
- Add weights to top board until you find the perfect amount. Too much weight makes a hard, dry cheese; too little makes a crumbly, overly moist cheese. The weight and time is a vital portion of the cheese recipe.

Project 32:
Farmhouse Cheddar

Making cheese in the modern age is more about enjoyment than survival, but it does help build planning skills and patience, both of which are essential to emergency planning. Making cheese is not hard, but it does take a long time for your finished cheese to age properly (6–8 months). I love it because it was one of those projects that looked daunting, but once completed really increased my confidence as a DIY prepper.

Equipment:

- Cheesecloth
- Colander
- Thermometer
- Cheese press
- String
- Slotted spoon
- Large pot (stainless steel or unbroken enamel *only*—aluminum or cast iron will produce off taste in product)
- Large bowl
- Measuring cups and spoons

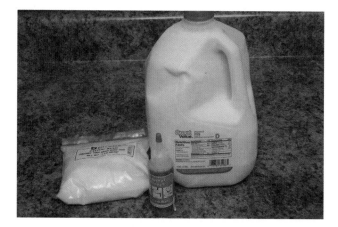

- Wooden cutting board
- Timer

Ingredients:

- 2 gallons milk
- 1 packet Mesophilic direct set culture (or 1 ounce of homemade)
- ½ rennet tablet dissolved in ¼ cup chlorine-free water
- 1 tablespoon cheese salt (or noniodized salt)

Directions:

- Heat milk to 90 degrees (goat milk to 85 degrees).
- Add culture, stir well, and let sit for 45 minutes while maintaining temperature.
- Add rennet by pouring gently through perforated spoon. Stir very gently to bottom of bowl for at least 1 minute.

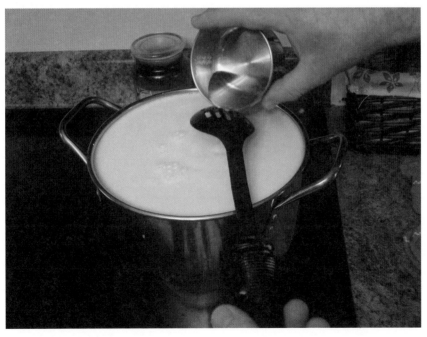

- You may also "top stir" the first ½ inch of milk for 1 minute to prevent cream separation if using goat's milk.
- Cover and let sit undisturbed for 45 minutes (until strong curd is formed).
- Cut the curd into ½-inch blocks.

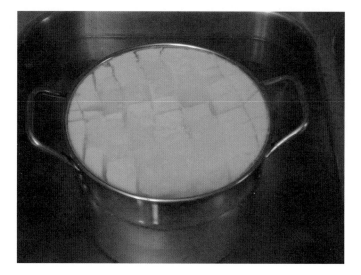

- Warm *very* gently to 100 degrees while stirring blocks gently. (Do this by placing pot into a sink of hot water and don't let the temperature of the pot rise more than 20 degrees every 5 minutes. As the curd heats and is stirred, the curds will separate from the whey and the curds will shrink.
- Remove from heat, cover, and let curds settle for 5 minutes.
- Strain the curds into a cheesecloth-lined colander (save the whey for ricotta and for baking—don't waste. . . .) Knot one corner of the cheesecloth around the other three to form a bag.
- Hang bag over pot for at least an hour.

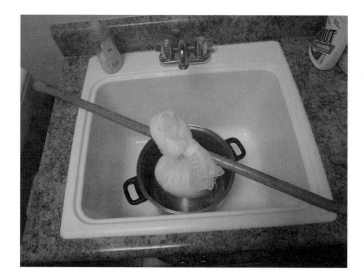

• Once the curds have drained, put them into a large bowl and mix with salt as you break curds into walnut-sized pieces.

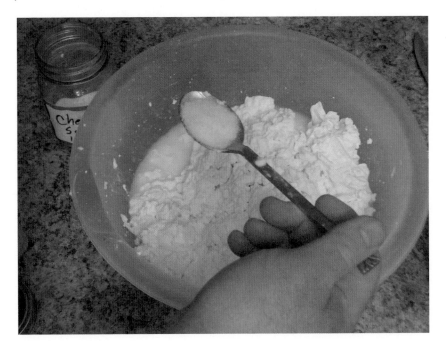

• Firmly pack cheese into a cheesecloth-lined mold; fold cheesecloth over top of curds. Any wrinkles in the cheesecloth will translate into divots and marks in your finished cheese.

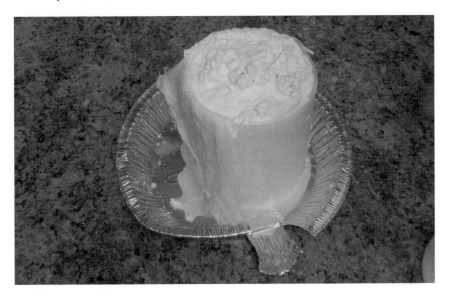

- Apply 10 pounds of pressure to mold for 15 minutes (whey will drain from mold).
- Flip mold and apply 20 pounds of pressure to other side of cheese for 12 hours.
- Turn cheese again and apply 20 pounds for an additional 12 hours.

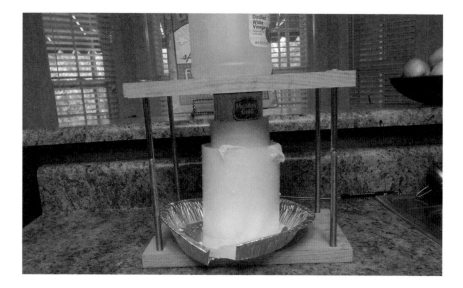

- Remove cheese from mold, and carefully peel cloth away, taking care not to rip cheese.
- Air dry the cheese at room temperature on a wooden board until a rind has developed (3 to 5 days). You must flip the cheese several times a day. as moisture will collect on board if you don't.

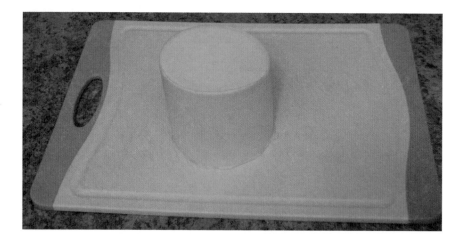

- Wax the cheese (or vacuum seal it) and age for at least 2 months –however, the longer it ages, the sharper it will be (6–8 months).

How to Wax Hard Cheese

Before refrigeration, making cheese was the best way to store milk. The aging times also killed any harmful bacteria that may have been present in the milk since pasteurization had not been discovered.

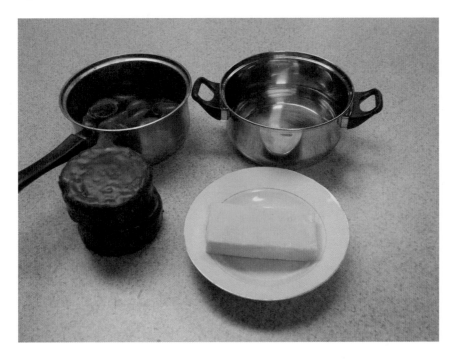

However, anyone who has left an open block of cheese in the refrigerator knows that air will dry out your beautiful cheese into an ugly yellow rock.

The process of covering the cheese in a protective coating of wax was created to seal in moisture and protect the cheese during aging. While my waxed cheese may not be the prettiest, it does its job at protecting my farmhouse cheddar until I can eat it.

The only wax you should use is cheese wax. Please do not use paraffin wax. Cheese wax actually melts at lower temperatures than paraffin, and it can reach a higher temperature than paraffin without catching on fire.

Be sure your wax is hot enough. Heat up your wax to 200 degrees so that when the temperature is dropped when you put it on the cheese, you still are applying wax that is 180 degrees or more.

Before waxing your cheese, either by putting your cheese in the wax or brushing it, be sure the cheese is completely dry.

Use several thin coats of wax instead of a few thick ones.

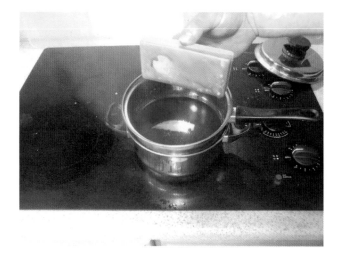

Hold the piece above the wax for a full 90 seconds to dry after you've dipped it before dipping in another portion of the cheese. If you lay it down to cool/dry, then you run the risk of a crack or crevice to be created while the wax is cooling. Also, don't allow the cheese to sit in the wax for more than 5 seconds when you dip it. You will run the risk of melting the cheese if you expose it to that heat for too long.

In case you are wondering, you can reuse your cheese wax. Just peel it, clean it with soap and water, and then you can remelt it and use it again.

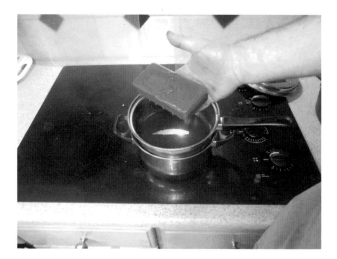

Project 33:
Recipe Mesophilic Cheese Starter

It seems like yogurt, cream cheese, sour cream, and a whole variety of cheeses use Mesophilic cultures to turn milk to cheese. It also seems like there has to be some way to make cheese without buying those little packages of powdered

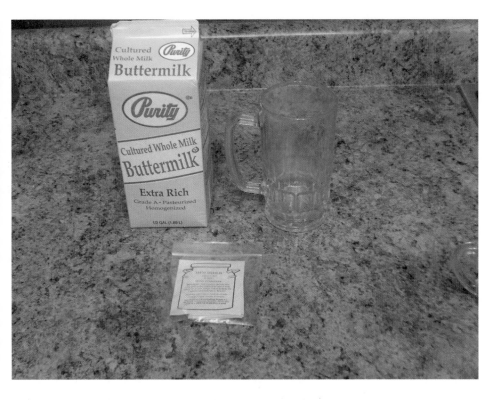

culture—I mean, we had cheese for thousands of years before we had big brown trucks to deliver the cultures.

I have been researching and found how extremely simple Mesophilic culture is to make at home.

This recipe uses a home freezer, but I heard of an anecdotal story of how some Eastern Europeans snuck their favorite yogurt cultures into the country through Ellis Island. It seems that the federal workers opened the jars of starter culture that our ancestors tried to import with them, smelled the yeastiness, and threw the jars out.

After this became known to those planning to immigrate, one particularly resourceful lady dipped several of her lace heirlooms in the culture and let it dry. The inspectors did not notice the bacteria dried on the cloth and when she settled in her new country, she simply dipped the lace in some warm milk and let the bacteria inoculate it.

Our process is a lot simpler. All you need is a measuring cup, an ice cube tray, and some cultured buttermilk.

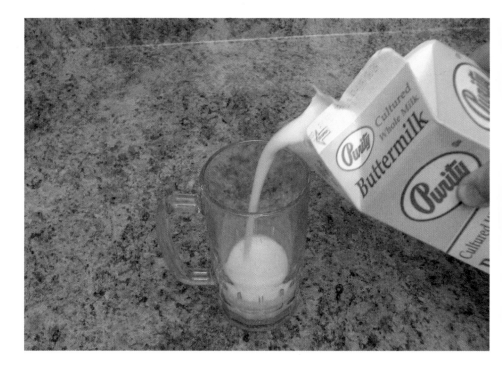

You see, cultured buttermilk contains a small amount of Mesophilic bacteria, just not enough to really get a cheese going, but if you set about 2 cups worth out in a warm room for 8–10 hours, the bacteria takes off and soon thickens the buttermilk and gives it a distinctive yeast smell.

If you take this thick buttermilk and pour it into a clean ice tray and freeze it, each cube is the equivalent of one ounce of Mesophilic culture.

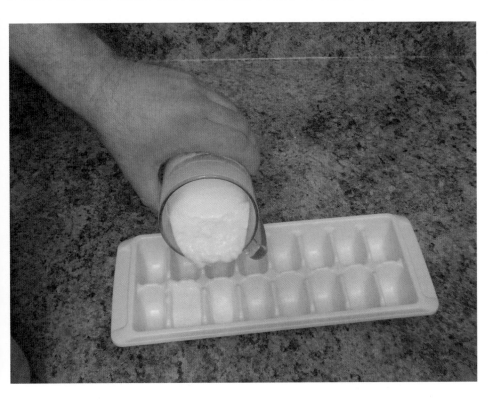

When you are ready to make cheese, simply drop one of these cubes in your milk and let it do its thing.

Just make sure to keep a couple of ice cubes back so you can use it to make more culture later. Once you get low you can just dump one of your culture cubes in some milk and let it sit until it has thickened.

Project 34:
Easy Homemade Wine

There are many reasons to make wine, from health to being cost conscious (or to make your own vinegars), but for me it's the experience of doing something on my own and freeing myself from reliance on a store for something I enjoy. This freedom soon translates into artistic license, because once you learn the technique and science behind wine making you are free to experiment and create wines from fruits and vegetables that you grow.

From a disaster prep standpoint, making wine has two good purposes, and you can decide upon the utility of them. The first is barter. If you put aside a bottle or two from every batch of wine you make, over the course of a year you will have a decent store of wine that could be traded for items you may not have. The second is that throughout history fermented beverages were served almost exclusively in place of water, as without modern infrastructure, it can become difficult for some to find safe drinking water. The fermentation process kills many harmful organisms, and the alcohol contained in wine serves as a good preservative.

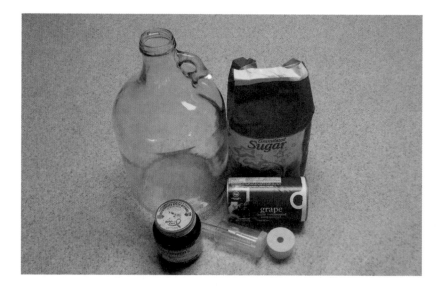

So for whatever reason you want to try to make your own wine, we will give you a simple beginner recipe that you can try before you decide to invest money in a better "quality" wine.

Equipment:

- 1 gallon jug, carboy, or bucket with a tight-fitting lid
- Airlock
- Funnel
- Rubber stopper
- Stockpot

Ingredients:

- 1 can 100% grape juice concentrate, thawed (get a brand without sulfides if you can, as they inhibit fermentation)
- 1 pound sugar
- 1 gallon unchlorinated water (if using tap—it is best to let it sit out a couple of days)
- Wine yeast (You can, and I do, use bread yeast, but you will not get a uniform result, and the wine's quality may vary)

Procedure:

- Clean the container with hot water. It is vital that your fermentation container is clean and sterile. You do not want your juice to rot; you want it to ferment, so you must kill any bad bacteria. Remember, you cannot sterilize something until it is clean.
- Pour the can of grape juice concentrate into the bucket, (if using a carboy or jug you will need the funnel).
- Pour in enough water to make ¾ gallon of grape juice/water mixture.
- Measure ¼ gallon of water into a large stockpot. Heat over low heat and add the pound of sugar. Stir until the sugar is completely dissolved. Once this solution of sugar and water is completely dissolved, add the entire pot of water to your fermentation container.
- Measure 3 tablespoons of sugar into a small bowl. Add 1 package of wine yeast. Add ¼ cup hot water. I have used bread yeast and champagne yeast also. The alcohol content may be slightly different, and the fermentation times may change, but they will all work.
- It should take about 10 minutes for the yeast to activate. Once it has become "bubbly," pour the yeast mixture into the jug.

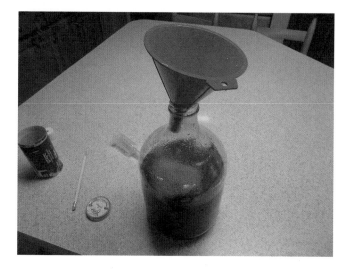

- Secure the airlock and rubber stopper on the carboy. Set the carboy in a spot where it will not be disturbed and the temperature doesn't have a lot of fluctuation. I keep mine in a bedroom we have turned into storage. It's close enough where I can check it, the temperature is stable, and I don't have to see it if I choose not to. I do make a concession to my bride—I keep the fermenter bucket in a big plastic container so in the event that any sloshes out it will be collected and not stain her carpet.

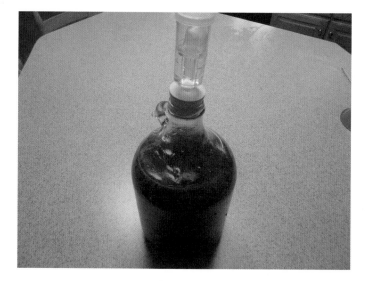

- Allow the wine mixture to ferment for approximately 1 month. When the airlock no longer bubbles when the jug or carboy is tapped, the wine is done.

Project 35: Tire Planters

I have to warn you, this can turn into a crazy passion. When researching this I saw many websites where people started using tires for planters and now own websites that sell tire art. I saw people making tire swings, recliners, rope horses, dragons, alligators, flowers, "Mexican clay pots," and even houses. After I built my first 4 planters I went back and got every tire the garage had and made about 9 more.

The basics are pretty simple.

- Find a used tire (I have found the larger the tire store the less likely they are to let you have any).
- Cut out the sidewalls.
- Flip it inside out.
- Paint it if desired.

I used a large hunting knife to cut. I have read about using jigsaws—and have been told that a wood blade with 10 or 11 teeth per inch is best. I have also been told that if you grind the teeth like you are making a knife (so the cutting end is very thin) and lubricate the tire with water as you cut it will be like cutting warm butter.

Either I was doing it wrong or that guy's butter was actually steel, because the jig saw did *not* work for me. A large sharp knife did the job pretty easily. More complicated did not make it easier.

You don't have to flip the tire inside out, but it makes it look less like a tire and takes a lot less paint (due to the tread). It's pretty simple—some tires flipped inside out so easily that I thought I was an expert—others took several minutes and more than one 4-letter word.

To flip a tire inside out, press down on one side and lift up on the other and try to flip the side of the tire that is away from you over the side near you and then down.

Basically, this is one of those things you have to do to understand, but it is really simple once you do it.

I then found the nice sunny areas I wanted planters and lined everything up because I will not move it once I have filled it. I found it took one wheelbarrow

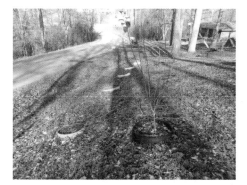

of dirt to fill each tire—but that depends on the size of tire and how compacted it is.

Many nice things about tire planters are that because of the black rubber they absorb heat well, so you can start your plants early. You get all the benefits of raised beds. They are easy to mow around as the mower bounces off of the tire. You are upcycling by taking something that takes a lot of room in landfills and turning it into something better. I have seen people selling tire planters for up to $30 (if you are willing to pay $30 for a used tire slapped with paint, call me and I will make you as many as you want).

I have read that some people are concerned with toxins leeching into the dirt—I did a little research and found that the main thing that leeches off of *washed* tires is zinc—which is bad for some plants, but at reasonable levels is something humans need. I also learned that the zinc is released as the tire breaks down, which happens over about 30 years. So *for me* I am not concerned. If *you* are, then don't plant edibles in your tires.

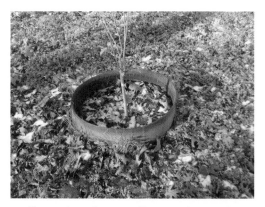

If you have a small tree that they can fit over, tires make great protectors.

Project 36: Planting Garlic

Generally, garlic is planted in the fall. This is because it needs a cold treatment to do well. If you have a long growing season like we do here in the South, you can get away with planting in late February or early March. If you wait that long your bulbs may not be as big as they would be if you timed it properly, but don't let that discourage you.

Each bulb has several cloves and each clove will produce a bulb, so each pound of garlic you plant will yield between 4 and 8 pounds of garlic at the end of the season.

You could go to the grocery store to buy garlic bulbs and break the cloves down to plant them, but if you do that you won't have any idea what type of garlic you are getting. You may introduce plant diseases into your beds.

When you break the bulbs down to cloves, you want to do it the day before or day of planting, but not any sooner because the cloves may dry out.

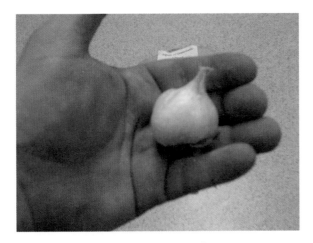

Inspect each clove and remove any that are tiny, have blue mold, or look dried out. You only want to plant firm healthy cloves.

Standard procedure is to make a furrow about 3 inches deep and place the cloves six inches apart along the furrow.

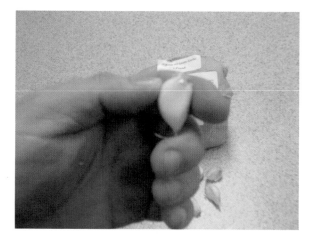

Be sure to plant the cloves pointed end up. If you plant them upside down, they will grow but will be misshapen and smaller than they should be.

Make your rows 10–12 inches apart. Rake soil back over the cloves so that they are covered by 2 inches of soil.

Project 37:
Pool Shock for Water Purification

Many campers use bleach for water purification, but bleach degrades over time, so it only has an effective shelf life of 6 months to a year. Dry High Test Hypochlorite (HTH) has no shelf life, and it's cheap—a 1-pound bag (which will purify about 10,000 gallons of water) is about $5. I spent a little more ($24) and bought a five pound jug (which is a *lifetime* supply) because it can be resealed.

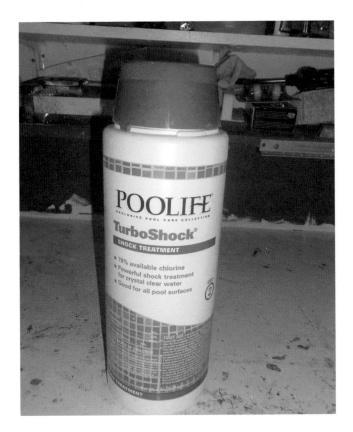

I will tell you, though, that this is not a perfect solution; this stuff is a powerful corrosive, and if you don't store this properly you *will* have problems.

- If it gets wet it will off-gas chlorine.
- It can corrode metals.
- If certain petroleum products mix with the HTH it can spontaneously ignite in a way you do *not* want to see.

Granular Calcium Hypochlorite

Only use HTH Pool Shock that does not have any algaecides or fungicides. Ingredients should read *calcium* hypochlorite and inert ingredients. Use a brand with at least 73 percent hypochlorite.

For this project I used Poolife TurboShock, but feel free to use any brand you wish as long as it fits the perameters above.

Before you begin mixing any chemicals in any way, please follow basic safety precautions. Make sure you do this in a ventilated area. Have plenty of water to dilute any mistakes. Wear eye protection for splashes. Lastly, always mix the powder into the water, *not* the other way around.

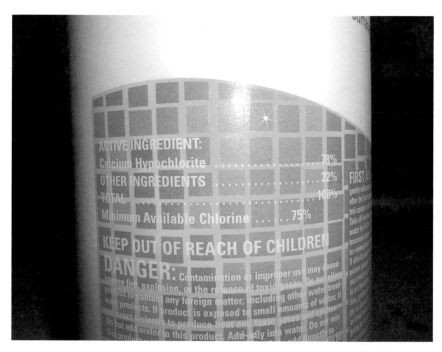

At least 73% Hypochlorite, and NO algaecide or fungicides

Add and dissolve one heaping teaspoon of high-test granular calcium hypochlorite (HTH) (approximately ¼ ounce) for each two gallons of water.

The mixture will produce a chlorine solution of approximately 500 mg/L (0.0667632356 ounces per US gallon), since the calcium hypochlorite has available chlorine equal to 70 percent of its weight.

To disinfect water, add the chlorine solution in the ratio of one part chlorine solution to each 100 parts of water to be treated. This is roughly equal to adding 1 pint (16 ounces) of stock chlorine to each 12.5 gallons of water to be disinfected.

To remove any objectionable chlorine odor, aerate the water by pouring it back and forth into containers to add air.

Chlorine Bleach

Common household bleach (unscented) contains a chlorine compound that will disinfect water. The procedure to be followed is usually written on the label. When the necessary procedure is not given, find the percentage of available chlorine on the label and use the information in the following tabulation as a guide.

Available Chlorine Drops per Quart of Clear Water

- 1 percent needs 10 drops
- 4–6 percent needs 2 drops
- 7–10 percent needs 1 drops

If strength is unknown, add 10 drops per quart of water. Double amount of chlorine for cloudy or colored water.

The treated water should be mixed thoroughly and allowed to stand for 30 minutes. The water should have a slight chlorine odor; if not, repeat the dosage and allow the water to stand for an additional 15 minutes.

Project 38: Bean Flour

Bean flour is one food storage option for those with wheat or gluten intolerance. It is also easier to grow beans than wheat, and gives you some variety in your food storage.

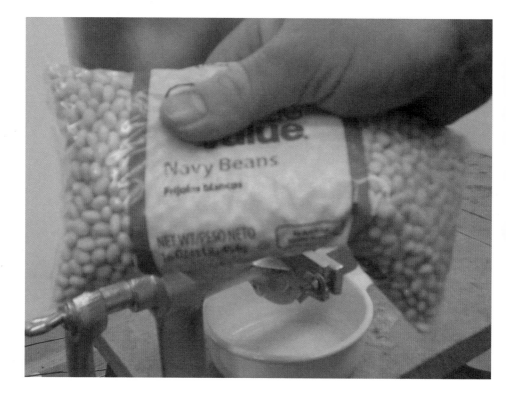

My first use of bean flour was in making some sourdough bread and substituting 2 of the 3 cups of wheat flour with 2 cups of bean flour made from navy beans.

There was little difference in the final product, but I did notice some subtle differences, especially in the dough. The bean dough seemed to have more bubbles formed and had a firmer, but less dense, texture.

You can replace up to one-fourth of the flour in any recipe with bean flour. Beans combined with grain form a complete protein, which is exceptionally efficient nutrition for the body, and best of all, no one has to know they are eating it! White bean flour or fava bean flour generally works the best for baked goods because it has a mild flavor.

Bean flour is also used to thicken or cream soups and stews. This is a great way to reduce the fat content of creamy soups. White bean flour has a neutral taste and a creamy flavor that could replace some of the heavy cream in vegetable soups. You can also use bean flour to make white sauce, as long as you use mild-flavored flour.

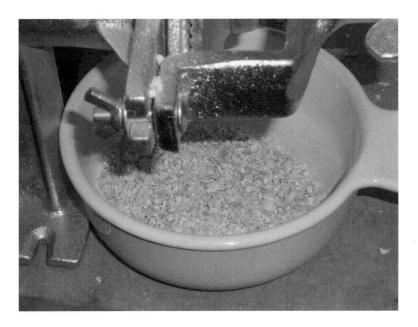

Whisk in bean flour to chicken stock, vegetable stock, or milk as a base for a fast, hearty soup. Be aware that the soup thickens in three minutes, so add any vegetables or meat before you add the flour. (Ratio is about 1:5, flour to liquid.)

There are several great recipes for using beans and bean flour for food storage, but today's project is to grind pinto beans into flour, and then use the flour to make "refried" beans.

Hopefully you have taken my subtle hint and bought a wheat grinder; if not, dust off the coffee can grinder and "grind" 5 cups of pinto beans into dust.

Once you have the bean flour you can use it in the very simple recipe.

Ingredients:

- 1 cup water
- 1 cup pinto bean flour

You can use 1 cup water to ¾ cup flour if you want a thicker texture.

Procedure:

- Bring water to a boil and whisk in bean flour.
- Cover and cook 5 minutes, stirring.

This recipe can be used in place of your "canned, refried beans" wherever it calls for refried beans.

Project 39: Recipe Vinegar

Making my own homemade vinegar was something I had been interested in for some time; however, I thought it was difficult. Turns out I was wrong.

Making vinegar is just as simple (if not more so) than making wine. Just as yeast eat sugar and excrete alcohol, acectobacter eats alcohol and excretes acetic acid (vinegar). They both need a warm, dark place to do their work. However, yeast works in an anaerobic environment; vinegar is formed in an aerobic environment. So keep your alcohol away from air, or it may turn to vinegar.

All you really need is a warm, dark place, a jug, some sort of alcoholic beverage (fortified wines, ports, and liquors don't work as well as wine or beers around 6 percent alcohol), cheesecloth or other means of keeping out debris while allowing airflow, and a mother (a starter culture of Acectobacter).

You can order a mother from several places online for 16 to 20 dollars, and generally they will be listed as either a red, white, or malt mother. The bacteria is the same; it's just in a different liquid. The reason for this is so you don't add a red wine–based mother in your pretty white wine and discolor it.

If you do not want to order a commercial mother, you can use apple cider vinegar as long as it is labeled "raw and unpasteurized"–hopefully you will also find the words "with mother."

Here is the procedure:

- Dump any leftover wine or beer (not both) into a crock, jug, or other stainless steel, ceramic, or glass container. (Aluminum, cast iron, or plastic containers will not work.)
- Dilute with a little water, no more than 50/50, and you want to leave room in the container for air to get in. The more surface area the faster your mother will grow. Also don't use tap water unless you give it time for the chlorine to evaporate (it will kill your mother).
- Dump in the mother—I made sure to get some of the chunks from the bottom of the Bragg's jar, but I don't think it is necessary. About one cup per gallon should work.
- Cap with a piece of cheesecloth held in place with a rubber band.

• Shake a little (again, probably not necessary).
• Store in a dark closet and come back in about 2 months.

You should have a leathery growth floating at the top of the liquid—that's a good thing, it's a healthy mother. If you don't then you may need to feed your vinegar with some fresh wine and a teaspoon or so of more raw vinegar.

If you have a vinegar crock with a tap near the bottom, once your vinegar has aged a couple months you can continually use it by tapping it as needed, and topping it off with whatever wine you have around as you open a bottle and don't finish all of it (if you're someone that does that—if I open something I tend to use it).

As one last caveat—if you plan on using this vinegar for canning, *please* invest in some acid test strips to ensure you have enough acetic acid to ensure safe food preservation. It may taste like vinegar but not be strong enough vinegar to kill the bad bacteria.

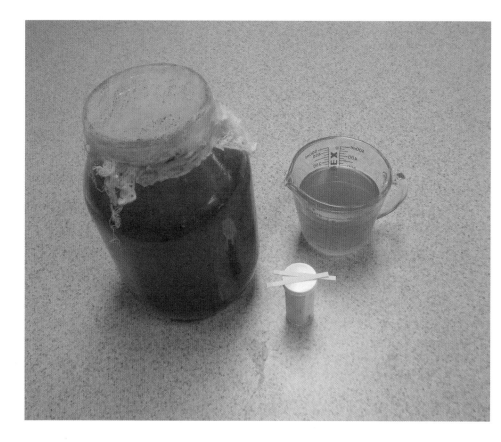

Testing and Refilling Homemade Vinegar

Once your vinegar has had time to steep, it's time to see about using it.

If you are going to use your vinegar for food preservation it must be at least a pH of 5.

The difference between pressure canning and boiling water canning is high or low acid foods—this cutoff is a pH of 4.6. Anything less than a pH of 4.6 is considered a high acid food.

Botulism cannot reproduce at a pH of 4.4 or less *but* remember, that the food you can, as well as the moisture from it, will change the pH by diluting your pickling solution.

To test, pour out a sample, stick a test strip in the liquid, and then compare it to the picture on the jar. The set of strips is a reasonable cost—around $7 for a jar full of strips.

However, you need to know that the FDA doesn't allow commercial canneries to use pH paper to test both because comparing colors is relatively subjective, and that the accuracy can degrade over time.

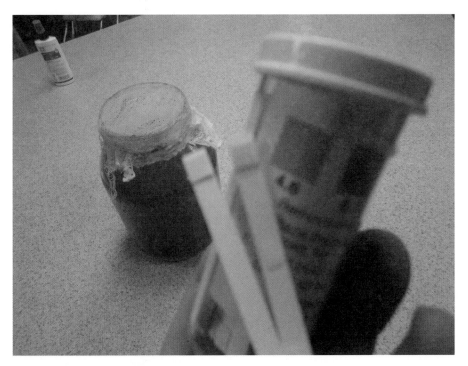

This vinegar was "off" the chart

I store my vinegar in brand new plastic milk jugs (HDPE #2); the rest was topped off with "fresh" wine and left to feed.

Many folks that make their own vinegar have one continuously fed batch—as they use it, they refill it. That is basically what I do; as I use mine, I just top it off with whatever leftover wine I have around.

In a perfect world, you should feed your vinegar regularly, as it needs the alcohol from the wine to keep the culture strong. In one of my recent batches my mother collapsed and sunk to the bottom because I only fed once when I began making the vinegar. Once it ate all the alcohol it basically went dormant.

The batch brewing right now (about a month later) has a much stronger, thicker mother floating on the top of the wine, because I have been adding about a cup or so of wine every couple weeks.

My plan is to filter and bottle my vinegar as I get full gallons worth. That's mostly because I have a case of milk jugs from my honey adventures and realized how long it will take me to fill 40 gallon jugs of honey from 4 hives (and how much slower gallons of honey sell compared to pints).

Making vinegar isn't really all that hard, and it is so much more fulfilling to cook with vinegar I made from wine I fermented from fruits I grew. . . . It may just be me, but mustard made from my homemade vinegar is so much tastier than store bought.

Project 40:
Recipe Sourdough Bread

If you are going to store wheat, you had better learn to use it. Since baking is an acquired skill, I want to share a pretty simple recipe, but the originator used measures by weight and I use it by volume to make it simpler.

This is not the most sophisticated recipe, but it works and I like the taste of this bread.

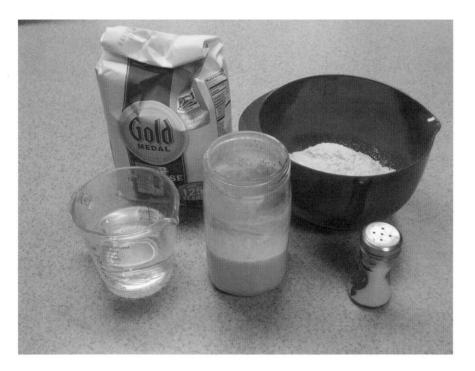

Ingredients:

- 1 cup water
- 1 cup Starter
- 2 teaspoons salt
- 3 cups flour

Procedure:

- Add starter to the water and mix.
- Dump in flour and salt and mix until you get one big ball of dough.

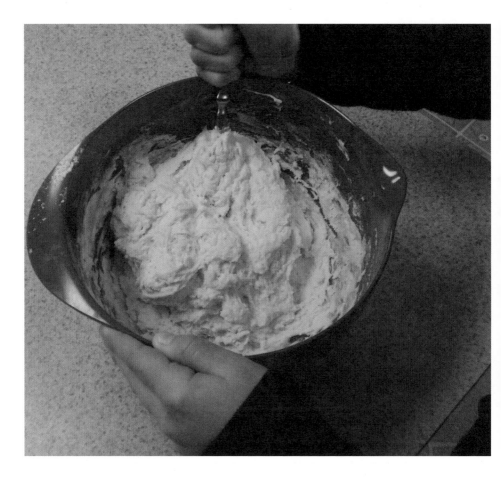

- Cover the bowl and let rest (I normally go 8 hours but have done it with significantly less time).
- Carefully use a spoon to help dough ball fall out of the bowl and onto a floured board or countertop.
- Stretch and fold the dough once by stretching dough into a rectangle and folding the sides together, and then the top and bottom in toward center.
- Place in oiled container (straight sided is best).
- Cover and let rise in 75- to 80-degrees Fahrenheit area for a couple hours or until it doubles in size.

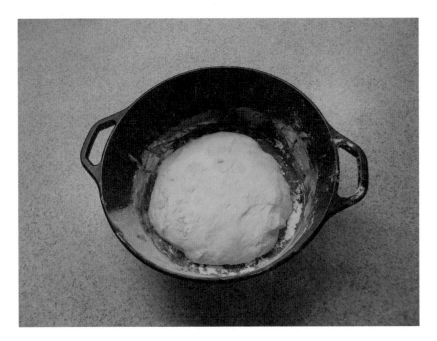

- Preheat oven to 425 degrees.
- Bake for 15 minutes. Keep an eye on this and use more or less time depending on your oven.
- Cool on rack.

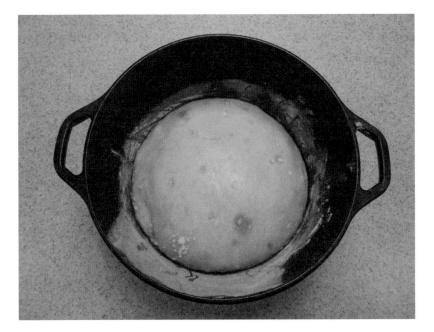

Project 41:
Antibiotic Garlic Tincture

Garlic has several reported health benefits, such as antibacterial/antibiotic properties, antiviral and antifungal benefits, it is an antioxidant, a natural mosquito repellent, and some believe it can help fight circulatory diseases.

While I am not a doctor, I have successfully used garlic tinctures to fight my chronic ear infections and to relieve colds.

One of the great chemicals in garlic is a powerful antibacterial agent called allicin. Since allicin is only present shortly after garlic is crushed and before it is heated, eating fresh garlic is best for treating a cold or flu. Some experts even recommend eating a clove or two every couple of hours until the bug is entirely gone. If you want to go this route, drinking milk as you chew the garlic will do much to prevent garlic breath.

However, you get more flexibility if you make a tincture of garlic, then you can take it internally, or use it topically as well.

As always, please consult a doctor before using any homeopathic remedy.

Ingredients:

• Ethyl alcohol (vodka, pure grain alcohol, white rum, or white whiskey)
• OR
• Vinegar (I prefer to use unfiltered organic with the mother)
• Garlic

Equipment:

• Mason jar
• Funnel
• Straining bag or cheesecloth
• Tinted glass jar with airtight lid
• Blender, food processor, food mill, or mortar and pestle

Procedure:

• Chop the Garlic
• Put twice the amount of vodka or vinegar as garlic into the mason jar

---

If dried garlic is used instead of fresh use a 5:1 liquid/garlic ratio instead of 2:1 for fresh. Either way, the garlic should be covered with liquid throughout the process of making tincture.

• Screw the lid on the jar tightly and shake it.
• Allow the garlic tincture to rest in the jar for 2 weeks to 1 month.
• Shake the tincture daily.
• Strain the garlic from the liquid.
• Store in the tinted glass; light will affect the quality of the tincture and may turn it a nasty gray/green color.
• Tinctures last several years when stored in a cool, dark place.

Garlic tincture can be used externally for the treatment of viral skin infections (athlete's foot), wounds, or ulcers. Garlic tincture can also be used as a natural remedy for flu, viruses, strep, worms, respiratory ailments, high blood pressure, colds, kidney problems, bladder problems, or earaches when taken orally.

Adults can take as much as a teaspoon 4 times per day orally.

Project 42:
Homemade Jerky

One of my favorite foods to make in my dehydrator is beef jerky. I don't make it as much as I would like though, because I have this uncontrollable impulse to sit down and eat it right after I make it. I do squirrel some away

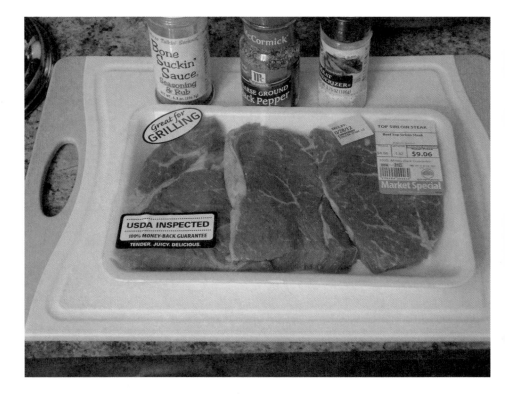

for storage but most of it gets eaten a small bit at a time as I walk through the kitchen.

It's a pretty simple process—select meat, trim, cut, season, dry, and store or eat it. Historically almost every culture has done it for food storage, and it remains a popular activity among outdoorsmen.

I like using sirloin, but any lean roast will do. You do not want a lot of fat, as that contributes to spoilage, so you also have to trim any fat you find.

Here's a tip for those that like jerky, but don't want to spend a lot on meat, or don't like slicing it. You can use prepackaged "steak-ums" or any discount cheese steak–type sliced meat. I have gotten them in bulk at the big-box grocer for around $1 a box on occasion.

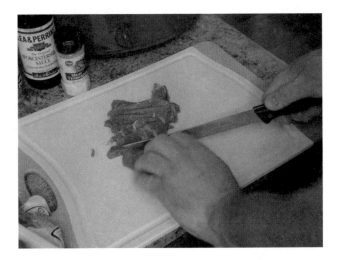

Slice your meat thin, around 1/20 inch thick. If you don't have a slicer you sometimes can get your butcher to do this; however, I have noticed that grocery store butchers are becoming less available as food sales change.

Personally I bought a hand crank slicer from an online auction, but I would also like to buy an electric one in the future. You can slice the meat against or with the grain, depending on your preferences; however, if you cut the slices against the grain it will be easier to chew and break up if you're going to make pemmican.

The next step is to marinate your meat for flavor. There are many recipes online and in print as well as premade marinades. Personally I throw together whatever looks good in the cabinet and mix with water. I use garlic powder, pepper, onion powder, and taco seasoning as a base of dry ingredients. If I am going to try to store it long term I use sodium nitrate cure to help with mold, but if I'm going to just enjoy it as is I leave it out. My wet ingredients are normally hot sauce, meat marinade (Dale's usually, but Worcestershire or soy

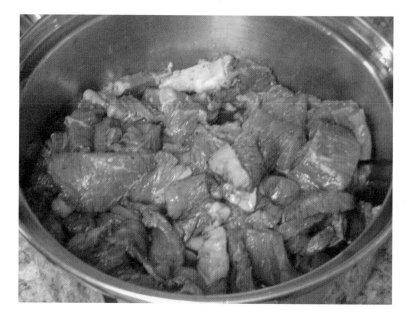

on occasion), wine, and sometimes vinegar (for a biltong flavor). This is all to my taste; feel free to experiment. I make enough mix to completely cover the meat to prevent browning (oxidation) and then keep it in the fridge for no less than 10 hours, but sometimes up to 24.

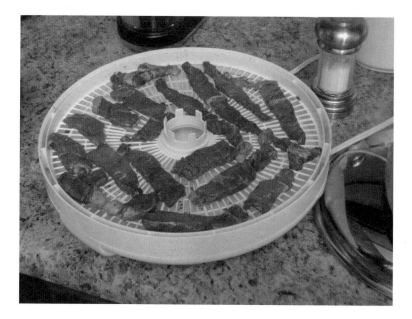

You can then coat the meat in a dry rub, but I normally don't as I use a lot of flavorings in the marinade and I don't want to overpower the meaty goodness of the jerky itself. You must be cognizant of the fact that dehydrating will concentrate the flavors so a lot of spice can quickly turn to too much spice.

You then need to remove the water from the jerky. I have an inexpensive round dehydrator as I collect the skills to build a much larger solar dehydrator, but you can use an oven on low (or around 160 degrees F) with the door cracked. You could make a cardboard box with a lightbulb and some sort of cheesecloth or mesh screen (be careful for the fire hazard). American Indians

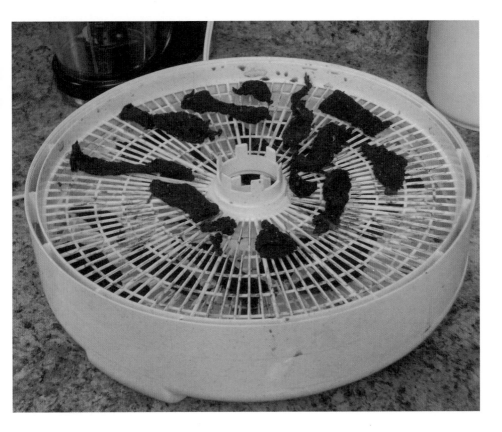

sometimes just draped the slices over teepees of sticks placed in the sun. It's not a hard process, but for food sanitation purposes I like using a method that

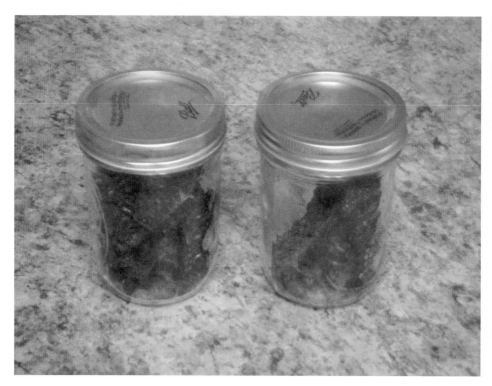

That entire package of steak fits in 2 small mason jars.

prevents flies from laying eggs, and produces enough heat to bring the meat's internal temperature to 160 degrees Farenheit without cooking the meat.

The drying process can last from 2 hours to 10 depending on meat thickness, humidity, and drying method.

If you want to store your jerky let it cool before sealing, so that any heat does not allow moisture to collect inside your container. Use mason jars to prevent additional moisture buildup and be careful about mold growth. (If you use jerky cure sometimes you can get a white bloom of nitrite crystals, so make sure any spots are that and not mold.)

Project 43:
One Brick Forge

I started by needing to make some tools for my new foundry and decided to "blacksmith" some from some bar steel I bought. I used my propane torch to heat everything up, but that was slow going and not very satisfactory.

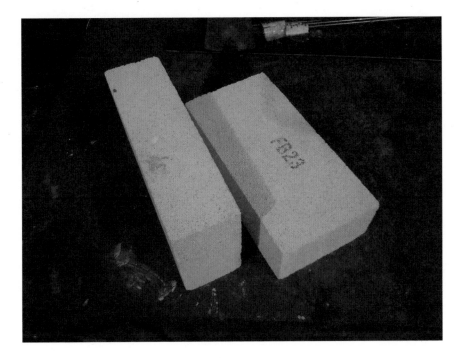

The basis of the forge is a single soft firebrick. I found one at the local ceramic supply store for $5. Soft firebrick is very light and crumbly—almost like an airy Styrofoam, which is what makes it perfect for this use.

All you need to do is to take an old 1-inch spade bit and drill out the center of the brick along its longest axis. Next turn the brick on its side and drill a hole halfway through the brick until you meet the hole you just drilled.

If you take a MAPP gas or propane torch and place it just outside the hole in the side of the brick and allow the flames to lap around the inside of the brick the center of the forge will get very hot. It will heat any metal placed inside the long drilled out hole to cherry red in just a few minutes.

The only problem is that the porous structure of the brick tends to hold moisture and if you get it hot very quickly it can crack. In his book, *Wayne Goddard's $50 Knife Shop*, Mr. Goddard suggests wrapping iron wire around the brick to hold it in place even if it cracks. I went a little overboard since I just got my welder. I welded up an angle iron box, inserted the brick, and then welded it shut. It was the first thing I welded that actually looked like a decent weld.

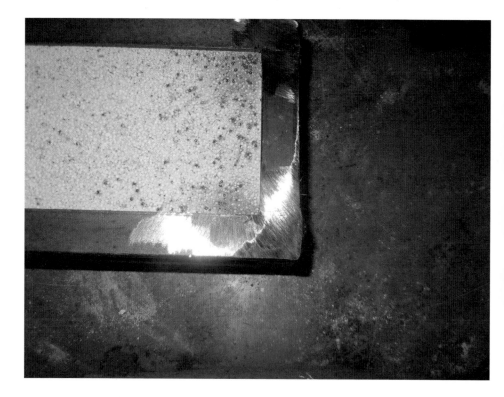

This forge works great for small pieces and I have used it a lot with no problems. It's a great piece of equipment to have in your shop.

Project 44:
Recipe Gluten Wheat Meat

My search to find alternative food sources has lead me to find seitan—which is basically the protein portion of wheat that has been flavored to mimic the taste of meat. You might not be familiar with the name, but if you have ever had mock chicken, beef, or pork at a Chinese restaurant, you have had seitan. Making it is pretty easy, but to the uninitiated it looks a little gross. In its

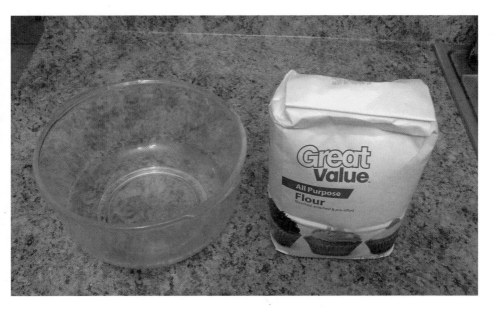

cooked, but not finished, form my wife wanted to throw it away, but cut up and put in chili, she doesn't know that she's not eating chicken.

Making it is simple; you basically make dough out of flour and water. Once the dough is made you rinse out the starch leaving a stringy mass of wheat gluten. You then add flavor by simmering it in broth and *bam*—you have a passable meat substitute.

Ingredients:

- 5-pound bag of flour—any flour, but the more gluten the more seitan you will get
- Lots of water
- Flavorings—I used chicken broth, garlic and herb powder, soy sauce, Dale's meat marinade, and a large onion.

Equipment:

- Large bowl
- Colander
- Crockpot

Procedure:

- Dump the flour in the bowl and add water to make dough. Add water in a little at a time because you do not want to make a paste.

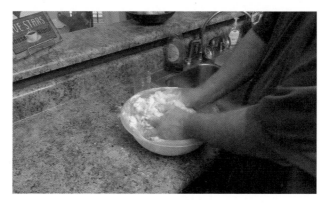

- Once it is kneaded into a single solid ball, cover with water and let soak for 20 minutes or so. The water should be a little milky.

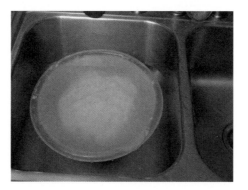

- Next, knead the dough a little under the water; the water should get very milky. That's the starch separating out.
- Drain into a colander and start running water over it. The water should be lukewarm and not under a lot of pressure. You want to gently rinse the starch away rather than blast it apart. Knead the dough under the water and watch the dough change consistency.

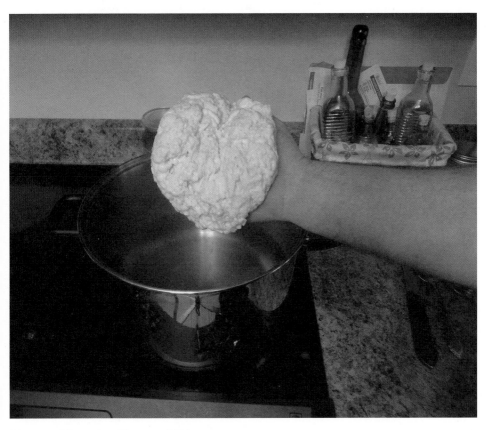

Rinse and knead until you get this.

- The dough will become stringy and stretchy, and I thought it looked a lot like brains. . . . But this is how you want it to look.
- Keep kneading until the water runs clear and it's one solid mass.

At this point you need to cook your gluten. Flavorings are up to you; you can use stock or Italian seasonings, or even sausage seasonings. I saw a cool recipe for seitan pepperoni that I am going to try one day.

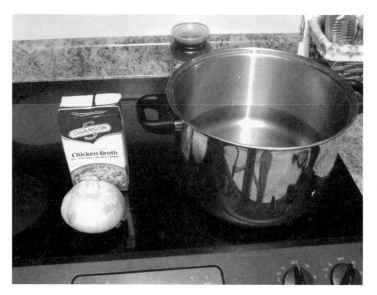

Flavor your wheat.

Some boil the seitan until it floats, but for ease I used a slow cooker. I simply dumped in a jar of canned stock and one onion, along with whatever cool seasonings I had in the cabinet. I cooked on high for about 2 hours and then left it on low for the rest of the night.

Right now it's in my freezer, but this weekend I am going to thaw it, cube it, and then dehydrate it for later use in white chili.

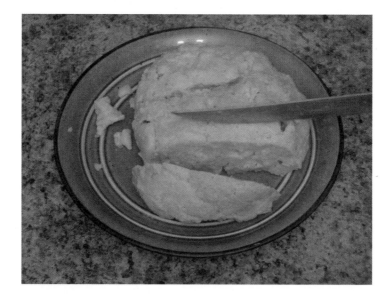

It's not brain surgery or rocket science, it's just a little messy kneading all that dough, but hey, if I can do it, you can too!

After a couple days in the fridge, I sliced a ½-inch slab from the ball and fried it with barbeque sauce. I then broke it into chicken nugget–sized chunks and stabbed them with a metal skewer and left them where the wife would find them. . . . She thought it was pork BBQ and said it was really good (though she did gag a little when I told her it was the wheat "brain" I made the weekend before). It tasted like a McRib from McDonalds (which it was probably pretty close to it).

I cubed the rest and dehydrated for chili later. This stuff has no taste to speak of, but it does have a "meaty" texture. It's kind of cool in a weird sort of way.

Project 45:
Making a Simple Knife from an Old File

If you do an Internet search on beginning knife making you will find a variety of articles on making a knife from an old file, and although this is probably one of the easiest ways to get started in knife making, I want to point out that historically, a file is much more valuable than a knife. It was not until rather recently that files became disposable; actually, older handmade files are thought by many to be much better than the machine-made files of today.

To make a knife you need to have steel with enough carbon to harden, but hardening brings brittleness, so you need to have steel that can harden enough to hold an edge but not become too brittle. The best solution is to buy known steel, but that is not always the DIY solution.

Procedure:

• Anneal the file to make it soft enough to work. Annealing alters the structure of the steel to make it workable. In a hot campfire or something like our one-brick forge, heat the file until it is glowing yellow-orange, then let it cool slowly (at its own pace).

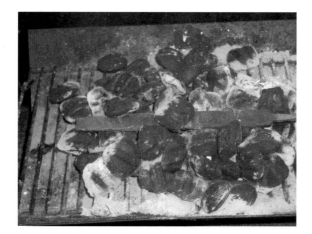

- Sand, cut, and grind the file to the shape you want. If you use a grinder take care not to go too fast and heat the metal up. I hold the knife in my hands and if it starts to get hot, then I know to slow down. Don't try to get a "sharp" edge; just grind down the blade to a 15-degree angle so that it is close to being sharp.

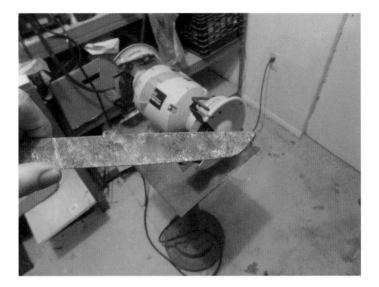

- There are several ways to attach a handle, but drilling two rivet holes, and riveting handle material to the tang is easiest for a beginner, make sure you drill the holes before you reharden the knife.
- Once the knife is shaped you need to harden it by heating evenly. You can use your brick forge, if you can fit the whole knife in it, but I like using a charcoal fire. I like using natural hardwood charcoal, as it has less additives that tend to add to scale on the knife blade. Heat to a light orange (20–30 minutes on a charcoal fire). Force air into the fire to supercharge it—watch the knife carefully and when it reaches a light yellow-orange color and seems a little translucent pull the knife out of the fire and check it with a magnet. When the metal is nonmagnetic quench the blade.
- Wearing thick leather gloves, and with a bucket of used motor oil quench the blade by evenly, yet quickly, lowering the blade vertically into oil. Stir the oil with the blade until the flames go out. Rest the blade against the inside of the oil container and wait until it is cool.
- Once the blade is cool check to ensure the blade did not warp. If it stayed straight, clean and sharpen the blade.

- Temper the knife by using a propane torch to slowly and evenly heat the spine of the knife to a yellow-brown "wheatish" color. Do not overheat the metal.
- Cut out two slabs of whatever handle material you want to use; oak works well.
- Rivet the slabs to either side of the knife and then sand and shape the handles to your desire. (You could also use epoxy to bond the handle to the tang of the knife for a more permanent bond, but it is not strictly necessary.)
- Enjoy your knife.

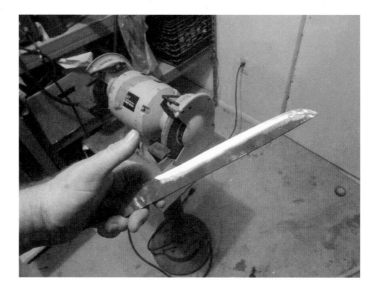

Project 46: Recipe Tofu/TVP

This project is very similar to the cheese making from earlier projects.

Basically tofu is a bean curd made by coagulating soy milk and then pressing the resulting curds into soft white blocks. It's very similar to making a vinegar-based cheese like ricotta.

To make tofu you only need soy milk, a coagulant, a pot, spoon, and sieve, and a way to press out the water. I used my cheese mold, but you could use a saucer pressing down on the curds in your sieve.

There are three basic types of coagulants: salts, acids, and enzymes. Enzyme tofu production is beyond my scope as a home chemist so I won't discuss it. I have also read that a lot of the medical problems some attribute to tofu stem from the use of enzymes but I am not a doctor, so you should research that yourself.

Salt Coagulants

- Calcium sulfate (gypsum) is the traditional and most widely used coagulant to produce Chinese-style tofu. It produces a tofu that is tender but slightly brittle in texture. The coagulant itself has no perceivable taste. Use of this coagulant also makes a tofu that is rich in calcium.
- Magnesium chloride (nigari) salts or calcium chloride (lushui) are the coagulants used to make tofu with a smooth and tender texture. In Japan, a white powder called nigari, which consists primarily of magnesium chloride, is produced from seawater after the sodium chloride is removed and the water evaporated.
- Magnesium sulfate (Epsom salt) is readily available and cheap, so for the beginner or first time user, this is a great coagulant to use

Acid Coagulants

These can affect the taste of the tofu more than salts, and vary in efficacy and texture. But the two most used are:
- Vinegar (acetic acid)
- Lemon juice (citric acid)

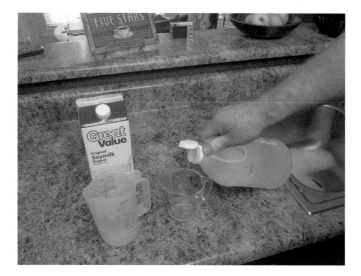

The recipe I used called for acid and it said either distilled white vinegar or lemon juice could be used interchangeably. I used vinegar.

Instructions:

- Boil your soy milk. The original recipe I started with (Rita Bingham's *Country Beans*), did not give a quantity, so I experimented and got good results with a half gallon. It said stir frequently, and I concur. I did not stir frequently enough and filled the kitchen with a nice chocolate smell as some of the soy milk scorched.
- Once it is boiling simmer for 7 minutes (stir frequently).

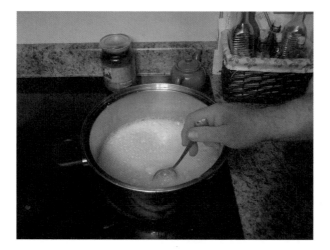

- Mix 1 ½ cups of hot water with ½ cup of acid.
- Once the milk has simmered remove from heat and stir in ⅓ of your acid into the milk. Stir very thoroughly.
- Keep the spoon in the pot and stop stirring. This sets up eddies in the milk to ensure a good mixing. When the milk stops moving, remove the spoon and sprinkle the second ⅓ of the acid on the top of the milk.
- Cover the pot and let sit for 20 minutes.
- Check the milk. It should curdle and the liquid should be clear but yellowish. If the milk has not fully separated add the last ⅓ of the acid, stir, cover, and let sit another 3 minutes or so.
- You will most likely need all the acid, but the more acid you use the more you will taste it, so by adding it in steps you may reduce the amount you will need to use, resulting in a purer product.
- Ladle the curds into a sieve lined with cheesecloth.
- Lift the edges of the cheesecloth and lift the bundle out of the sieve and place it into your press.

The weights and press times will change depending on how firm you want your tofu. Ten minutes with a quart mason jar of water will give softer tofu; double the weight and time for a firmer tofu. I used a quart jar of honey and 20 minutes and it turned out pretty good.

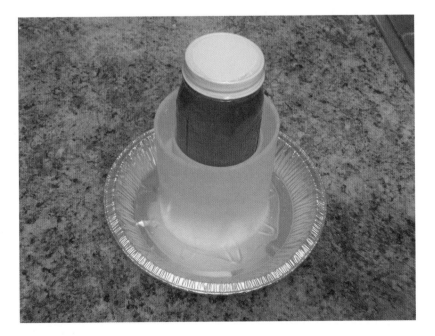

Once it has been pressed, place the tofu in a bowl of cold water for everything to set.

Tofu tastes best a few hours after it's been made. If you make your tofu in the morning, it will be at its peak at dinner.

If you will store the tofu for more than a day, cover the tofu with water. Since it is preservative-free, homemade tofu should not be kept more than a couple of days.

If you intend to eat the tofu on the same day, don't put any water in the container. Put on an airtight lid and store in the refrigerator until ready to eat.

Homemade TVP

Textured Vegetable Protein (TVP), also known as textured soy protein (TSP), soy meat, or soya meat, is a meat replacement or meat extender made from defatted soy flour (which is what is left after you squeeze out soybean oil).

It's popular in food storage because it is cheap, quick to cook, contains no fat, and has a protein content equal to that of meat.

Making TVP is an industrial process where hot soy flour is extruded into various shapes (chunks, flakes, nuggets, grains, and strips) and sizes. The defatted thermoplastic proteins are heated to 150–200°C, which breaks them into a fibrous, insoluble, porous mass that can soak up as much as three times its weight in liquids.

TVP can be mixed with ground meat to a ratio of up to 1:3 (rehydrated TVP to meat) without reducing the quality of the final product.

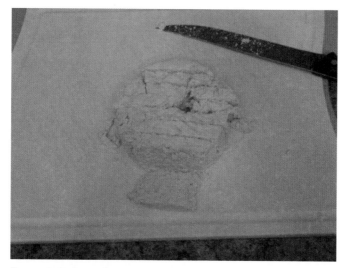

Frozen tofu is grainy.

TVP is primarily used as a meat substitute due to its very low cost at less than a third the price of ground beef, and when cooked together will help retain more weight from the meat by absorbing juices normally lost.

Now, this process is beyond my scope, but in doing research I figured if I can make tofu I surely can make TVP, so I searched until I found a recipe that gave me a workaround to make a product that is very similar in usage to real TVP.

I froze my tofu for 48 hours to give it a meat-like texture. I then let it thaw and once that was done, I simply crumbled it up. If I was making chili or burgers or whatever, I could then mix the thawed tofu crumbles with my meat. However, to make the TVP, I would need to dehydrate it.

In the dehydrator, the tofu dried very quickly and resembled the hamburger rocks I made a few months ago. The only difference was that the TVP was lighter in color and did not have a taste. However, that's a good thing, as the pores created in the freezing process will suck up the cooking water and make the TVP take on the flavor of whatever you a cooking it with.

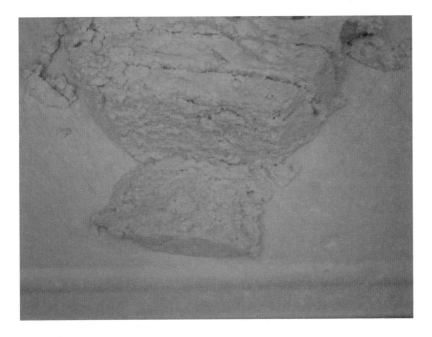

Project 47:
Homemade Desiccant for Long-Term Storage

Moisture is one of the largest threats to long-term storage, and over the years a variety of commercial products have been created to absorb moisture in gun safes and other storage areas.

I came across a unique homemade dessicant discovered during WWII as the Department of Energy at Oak Ridge experimented with devices to help with civil defense.

An engineer by the name of Cresson Kearny designed a homemade device used to measure radioactive fallout. This device used materials easily scavenged, and it included a homemade drying agent made by heating common gypsum wallboard (Sheetrock).

Do *not* use calcium chloride; use gypsum Sheetrock only.

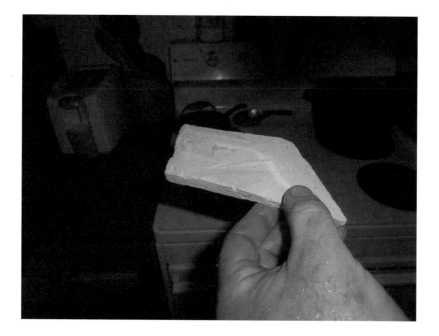

Instructions:

- Obtain a piece of ⅜-inch thick gypsum wallboard approximately 12 inches by 6 inches.
- Cut off the paper and glue (easiest done by wetting the paper).
- Break the white gypsum into small pieces no larger than ½ inch.
- Heat the gypsum in an oven at its highest temperature (which should be above 400 degrees Fahrenheit) for 1 hour.

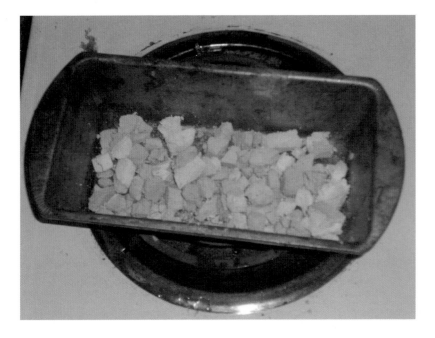

Heat the gypsum no more than two pieces deep in a pan.

Alternatively, you can heat the pieces over a fire for 20 minutes or more in a pan or can heat to a dull red.

- Anhydrite absorbs water from the air very rapidly, so quickly store in an airtight container while it is still hot. A mason jar is ideal.

Project 48:
Parabolic Solar Heater

I am a fan of solar energy, especially when its limitations are accounted for. Through research, I have decided that the heating aspect of solar is easier (and cheaper) to utilize than converting it to electricity.

In order to make the solar heater I dismantled an old DirectTV dish and sanded it smooth. I then painted it with black paint.

I cut strips of the mirror film and attached them to the dish. It's easiest to just cut straight strips and overlap them slightly. Early cartographers learned that it is impossible to draw a round Earth accurately on a flat sheet of paper; it's the same with the film and a parabolic dish. You cannot just slap the film to the dish; it will bubble up and refuse to form to the shape. Some try to calculate the curve and cut out "pie" slices, but this works best in theory; the math works, but it does not translate well to the real world. Strips that are allowed to slightly overlap each other work the easiest.

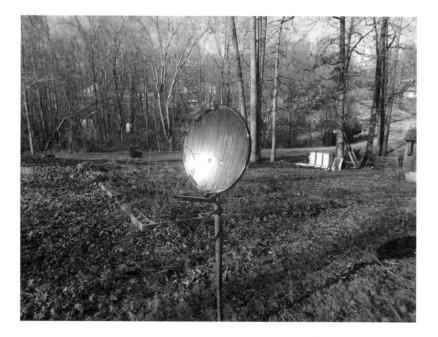

You will find it impossible to separate the thin strip of film from its backing by hand. However, if you attach a piece of tape to both sides of the film the backer will adhere to the tape, so when you pull the tape in opposite directions the film will peel away.

Very carefully install the film on your dish; if you have ever installed window tint, it is the exact same process. I started in the center and worked outward, as this was easiest for me. I imagine it does not make a big difference. Just try not to overlap the strips too much, don't allow bubbles to form, and don't get too worried about the holes for the mounting bracket.

After the strips filled the dish, I took a very sharp razor knife and cut a cross into the area of the mounting bracket holes. This allows the screws to be inserted back into the dish. I also trimmed around the edges of the dish.

I then reinstalled the dish on the post (don't just leave it there: the focused sunlight can be dangerous—so don't leave it unattended for long periods), pointed it at the sun, and rigged an empty glass jar at the focal point.

The sunlight then heats whatever is in the jar. You can use this to cook. I have seen this on a large scale to boil water and even make steam.

Project 49:
Lawn Mower Generator

I have long wanted my own generator, but a $500 and up price tag kept me from purchasing one new. After some Internet searching and sleepless nights I found a good tutorial online at http://www.theepicenter.com. What I liked best about the tutorial is that Brian at Epicenter has already worked out the kinks and sells the materials. I have no connection with Epicenter, and the only things I have bought from them were for this project, but what dealings I have had with them were fair and honest. Brian was also kind enough to let me copy some of his wiring diagrams for this project.

A coworker gave me an older Craftsman lawn mower for this project. I ordered the plate, an alternator, wiring harness, pulley, and two belts from the Epicenter website (approximately $160 with shipping).

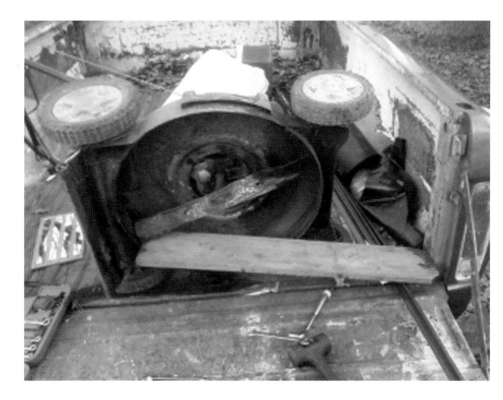

While waiting on the parts, I laid the mower on its side in the bed of my truck (being careful to keep the gas tank side up) and wedged a 2×4 between the truck bed and the mower blade to keep it from spinning while I unscrewed the blade. I did use some kerosene to loosen the nut (Liquid Wrench is almost pure kerosene).

I used a pulley puller to remove the blade from the shaft.

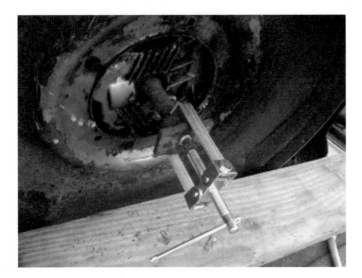

I purchased 5 bolts, 10 washers, 1 lock nut, and 4 1-inch spacers for about $15 to not only attach the engine to the plate adapter but also to align the pulley on the mower to the one on the alternator.

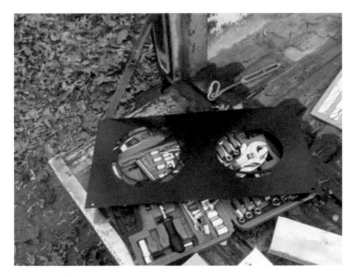

Once the plate arrived, I measured it and built a frame of scrap 2×4. The plate measured 12×24 so I cut two 2-foot lengths of 2×4 and 2 9-inch lengths. After screwing them together, it made a perfect frame.

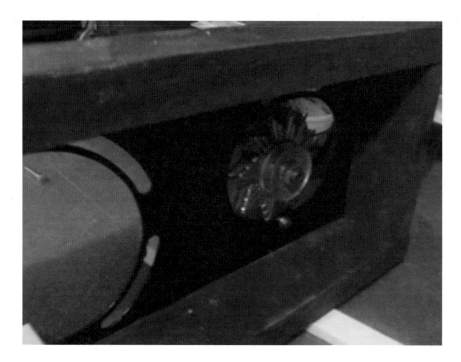

As soon as the paint dried I screwed the plate to the box and attached the alternator. It fits just like an alternator in a car. One screw fits in a whole in the plate, while a bolt fits in an adjustment slot in the plate and through the alternator and locks with a nut. To tighten the belt you loosen the bolt and move the alternator in the adjustment slot.

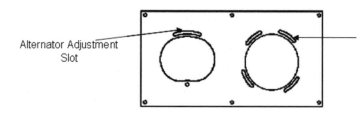

Alternator Adjustment Slot

These cut outs for the engine mounting bolts allow you to twist the engine to fit.

Plate Diagram Alternator cutout on left; engine cutout on right
(courtesy of theepicenter)

Next I installed the pulley on the shaft. I set in a ¾₆ keyway in the shaft and pushed the pulley onto the shaft. I used a dead blow hammer to knock it flush.

Once the pulley was installed and tightened, I installed the engine. The cutouts for mounting the engine were larger than my bolt heads, so I sandwiched the plate between two large fender washers; the spacers fit on the bolts on the top of the plate raising the entire engine over the frame. This is because the shaft is much longer than the alternator shaft.

Depending on the type of alternator you use and how it's regulated, there are different ways of connecting everything. I used an external switch and my alternator has an internal voltage regulator, so my wiring looks like the first schematic below.

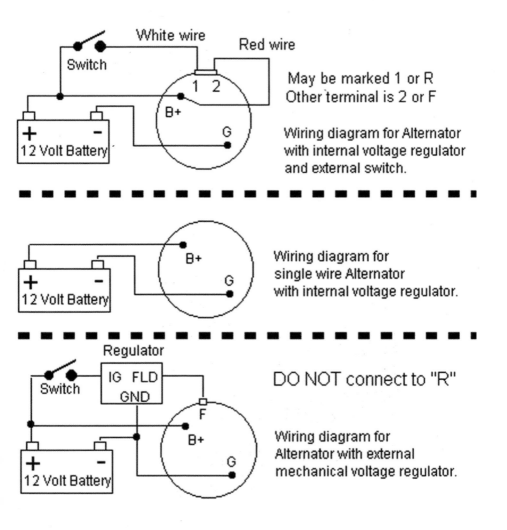

To keep things easy I paid an extra couple bucks for the wiring adapter for the alternator. You don't have to use Epicenter's alternator or their harness, but since I would have to either buy a new one or go to the junkyard and remove one on my own, I kept it simple and bought theirs.

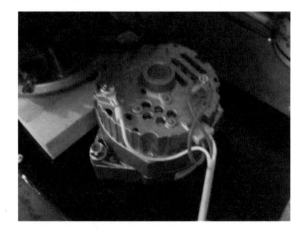

I used their adapter, some 14-gauge red and white wire, a 50 amp switch, some connectors, and heat shrink to rig up a wiring harness that snaps into the alternator. I probably should have used full battery cables to hook the alternator to the battery, but the run is short, the amps are low, and I will be next to the generator while it is running so I can monitor it if it gets hot.

Most lawn mowers come with a safety device that you must hold in order to keep the engine running. Mine was on the handle of the lawn mower. I looked at it and decided to keep it functional rather than safety wire it closed. What I

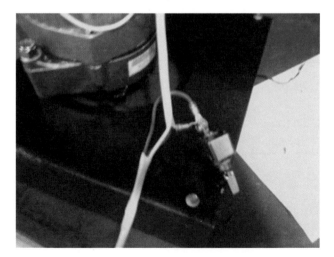

did was wire a washer to the linkage, which allows me to pull it tight and loop it over the linkage bracket. If I need to stop the engine quickly, I can just pull the washer off the bracket.

In order to use the generator, you must have a battery; this is because the voltage regulator needs to be energized to function. This generator is really just a souped-up battery charger, as the alternator's voltage regulator puts out the exact right voltage for charging car batteries. (Imagine that . . .)

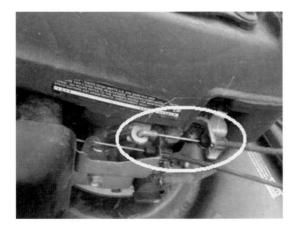

Some other things to consider are that because lawn mowers use light flywheels, they depend on the mass of the blade to idle correctly. So when choosing a pulley make sure you get a cast iron pulley with a little mass to it.

You do not have to use store-bought parts if you have parts at hand. I could have gotten by with using a piece of plywood as a base. If I had drilled a hole for the shaft to sit, I could have used the engine as a template to mark where to drill my mounting holes. This is a project for using your mind instead of your money to come up with a solution to a problem. I used more money than needed so I could spend less time considering solutions to problems of mismatched parts. Lastly, don't scrimp on the belt quality, and buy more than one. If you are relying on a generator you made from your dead car then it's a really *bad* day, and you probably aren't in a position to go to the auto parts store . . .

I really like this project; it's one of my favorites I have attempted this far. Since I cannot leave well enough alone, I plan on taking it a couple steps farther. The first major upgrade is that I plan on making a little switchboard to mount the throttle assembly and switch a little better. Next I plan on converting the carburetor to run on LPG gas from bottles, which will make the logistics of fuel storage safer while allowing me longer run times and faster refuels. I also plan on making a second lawn mower alternator combo, which I modify to make a welder. This is something 4X4 enthusiasts have done for years.

Project 50:
Recipe Pemmican

Pemmican is a mixture of dried and pounded meat and rendered fat. Since meat spoils rapidly it needs to be preserved, but because of the differences in makeup, meat and fats have to be preserved using different methods.

In pemmican, dried meat and rendered fat are preserved separately and then mixed back together to make a calorie-dense food that has a long shelf life. Traditionally we hear about pemmican being made with dried berries also, but that did not make up the bulk of pemmican creation until the Europeans began buying it that way.

Traditional Pemmican:

• Separate the meat from the fat.
• Dry the meat into jerky.

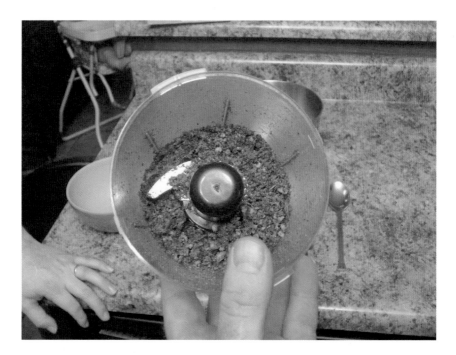

- Grind the meat. Use a commercial grinder or pulverize. I threw mine into a blender.
- Render the fat.
- Combine meat and fat, in a ratio of 2 parts meat to 1 part fat.
- Pack in airtight containers.

If you want to add dried fruit you can do that also.

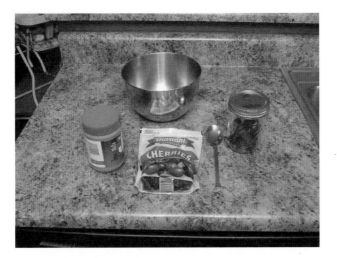

For a more modern pemmican (and easier to convince your wife to try) you can substitute peanut butter for the fat.

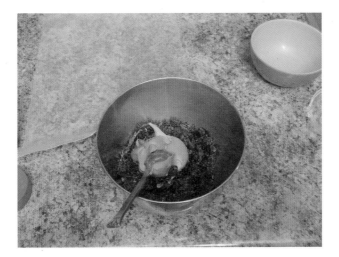

I dried a bag of freeze-dried assorted fruits and added it with the peanut butter and meat. My wife ate some and would do so again. I doubt she would if she saw me dumping in a jar of rendered fat though.

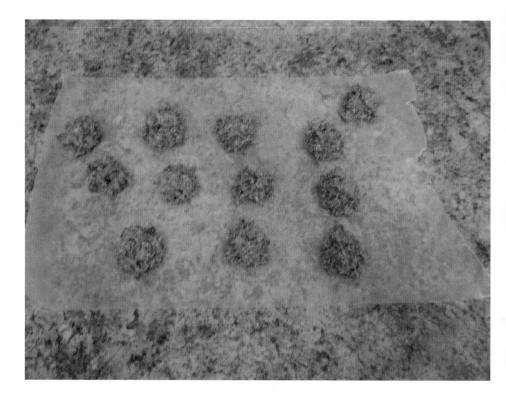

Just one caveat: this stores well and tastes pretty good, but it is very calorie dense so it's probably best suited as a meal replacement and not a neat snack.

These pemmican balls are also really good rolled in oatmeal, but once again, be warned that you can forget just how much protein is in a couple of these balls and eat them like snacks, when 4 or 5 of them would be a full day's ration.

Project 51:
2 Cycle Gas to Steam Conversion

This project has been one of my favorites so far. When I first saw this concept, I was a little overwhelmed. I thought it was magic and that anyone that could convert an internal combustion engine to work on steam had to be a genius. However, by the time I had enough projects under my belt to have the confidence enough to try it I found it to be simple.

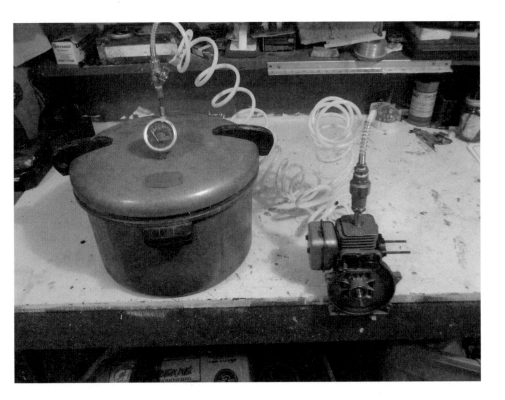

I need to say this upfront: This project used steam under pressure; therefore there is an element of danger to this. Steam engines cannot be safely run unattended. If you are going to build this or any other steam project you must use some uncommon sense and work carefully.

Now that the safety issue has been broached, I will address the question that my wife, mother, and coworkers who think I am crazy have asked repeatedly. That question is *"why?"*

Well, the most obvious answer is that I think it is cool, but what I tell my wife is that a steam engine gives me a redundant power source that does not need oil-based fuel. I can go out and cut wood and convert wood into electricity. While this is not as efficient as a purpose built steam engine and boiler or a wood gas system, it is much cheaper and simpler to build.

To make this project you need three components: a boiler, an engine, and a generator.

The boiler uses a salvaged Weedeater, but most any engine will work if you understand the process and can adapt to overcome. I used a Weedeater because it was free and the simplest to convert. You will also need a ¾ brass check valve, a pushrod, and miscellaneous plumbing bits and pieces.

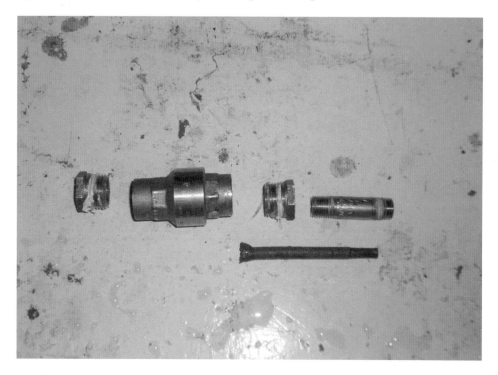

The idea is to create a single acting steam engine (meaning the steam only acts on one side of the piston) by using a pushrod inserted through the spark plug hole to push open the check valve when the piston is at Top Dead Center

(TDC) so the steam will push the piston down just like the gas explosion did when it was an internal combustion engine.

The first thing to do is strip your Weedeater down to bare block. Just start unscrewing stuff, but leave the internals alone.

You will need to keep the flywheel attached to the engine, as you will need the weight to return the piston to TDC. Otherwise the engine will quit. I plan on casting a new flywheel (formulas for this can be found in Steven Chastain's book on inverters and generators); I just haven't gotten to that yet. Once you get the block stripped down you need to find a pipe nipple that will screw into the spark plug hole.

Your check valve will screw onto the other end of the nipple, but first you need to take some measurements. You have to create a rod that is long enough to push the check valve open when the piston is at TDC. It should also be long enough to keep a portion of the rod in the pipe nipple so it does not fall into the combustion chamber, yet short enough to let the valve close as soon as the piston starts to move. If it is too long or too short the engine will either lock up or be hard to start.

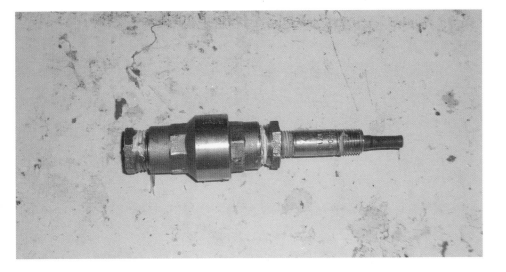

An easy way to measure would be to screw everything together and measure the exposed length of pipe (that way you don't have to keep track of the amount that is threaded). Unscrew everything and rotate the piston to TDC. Insert a rod to measure from TDC to the top of the spark plug hole. The last measurement is from the bottom of the check valve to its open position. You do this by taking your measuring rod and pushing the valve open. Add the three together and that should be the length of your pushrod. Personally, I added a tiny bit to the measurement to account for my problem with attention to detail, and then used a file to custom fit everything. I kept assembling the engine and rotating the crankshaft to check if it would open the valve and cycle smoothly. To make this simpler I used a piece of old ink pen shaft as my push rod, with the idea I would measure it when I got the dimensions correct and make a new rod out of a metal rod. In actuality, I just glued a carpentry nail inside the plastic shaft and am pretty pleased with the results.

The only other mechanics you will need to do to the engine itself is to adapt the top of the check valve to fit a steam line. I just screwed in an air chuck quick connect so I can use an air line, but I am sure you can use a metal line if that makes you more comfortable.

To start the engine you have to add the steam and then somehow turn the flywheel to start the process. I am not happy with this procedure, as I am afraid I may end up hurting myself when everything starts to move, but so far I haven't had any Tex Grebner moments . . .

To be quite honest, converting a steam engine in this manner is relatively cheap—even buying everything new, I am still around $50 with the $30 check valve being the most expensive part. It is also a lot easier than I imagined; however, learning about steam generation has caused me a lot of anxiety and has taken up the most time in this project.

Creating steam, especially under pressure, is dangerous. A mistake in this process turns into bomb pretty quickly, and a leak can actually melt your face off. Because of this I have decided to totally separate the boiler discussion.

Steam Boiler

First off, playing with steam—especially under pressure—is a dangerous thing. Failure to use common sense and a healthy set of caution can melt the flesh from your bones. However, if channeled properly steam can transmit a lot of power and turn heat to torque.

I have already shown you my Weedeater conversion to a basic single acting steam engine, now I will show my home workshop boiler. This portion of the project caused me the most sleepless nights and research, and I fully expect you to do your own research if you plan to create your own boiler. As I am not there to ensure you take the necessary precautions, I cannot be held liable for your actions.

That being said I used a pressure cooker for my boiler. I did this because I know it is tested to the pressures I plan on using for my boiler. I flirted briefly with a firetube boiler, but in the end, I felt more comfortable using something that was designed and constructed to boil water under pressure.

My pressure cooker (as well as every other cooker I have seen) has a pressure release that is designed to rupture well before the pressures inside the cooker endanger the integrity of the cooker itself. If this every goes off, cut the heat immediately and get *away*.

The pressure cooker has a pressure gauge on it also. The Agricultural Extension Office will test your gauge to ensure it is accurate (for food safety purposes). This calibration should be done annually, for food preservation, and I would suggest you get it checked *before* you modify your boiler, as I doubt they will test it with a roll of copper pipe coming out the end. They may even call the revenuer's thinking you have built a still. . . . (By the way, my boiler is aluminum, and that reacts with alcohol, so my steam boiler is in no shape, form, or fashion an alcohol distillation device.)

The other thing your pressure cooker should have on it is a weight of some kind to let steam out during the cooking process. This is the only thing of the three you should mess with. I used some tools and unscrewed it from the cooker lid. I replaced the weight with a brass ¾ mpt fitting and used hard copper line to attach the fitting to a ball joint and a quick-release coupling. (Before I use this for more than testing I will also plumb in a 150 psi safety valve.)

From the quick-release coupling I attached an air tool line—I looked into using soft copper ¼-inch tubing, and even though the burst pressures were

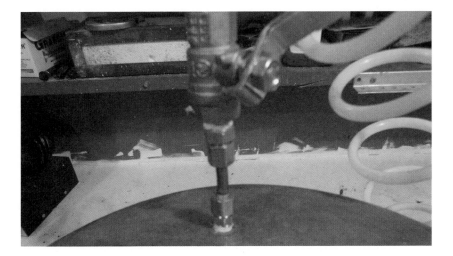

900 psi, which was plenty strong enough, for testing I wanted the flexibility of a hose.

When filling the pressure cooker/boiler do not overfill it. Don't go more than ⅓ full or you could have dangerous overpressure. Believe me, just a small amount of water will run Weedeater steam conversion for a long time, especially considering this is something you cannot fire and forget. If you heat your boiler you *must* be present at all times.

So in closing, a pressure cooker makes a pretty decent steam boiler, but you have to take into consideration the strength of all the components and realize that you are dealing with more extreme heat and pressure, and if a failure occurs it will be at the weakest link. You have to think through the process and ensure that precautions are taken to keep that weakest link in a safe place.

Project 52:
What Is EMP?

Electromagnetic pulse protection can be a contentious subject among preppers. In my experience there are two dominant views on faraday cages, and which camp you belong to depends on whether you are a ham radio operator or not. I base my ideas on the training I received when I worked as a radiological emergency response planner and the FEMA document CPG 2-17.

CPG 2-17 Volume I explains the science behind electromagnetic pulse (EMP) and the protection needed to mitigate this threat. Volumes II and III of the CPG series deal with the construction of protection devices, as well as show the reader how he or she can harden structures against electromagnetic pulses. Unfortunately, FEMA has discontinued the series, and the books are the "holy grail" of EMP documents, so they are extremely hard to find.

An EMP is a burst of electromagnetic radiation. Typically we think of EMP as coming from a nuclear explosion or from the sun. However, these are not the only situations where you can get an EMP. Several types of high energy explosions as well as suddenly fluctuating magnetic fields can produce EMP.

What you need to realize is that EMP is electromagnetic radiation, and as such fits in the electromagnetic spectrum. This is the range of all possible frequencies of radiation emitted. Light, heat, sound, radio waves, electricity,

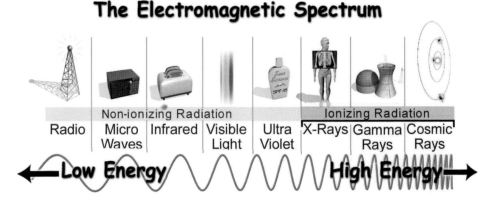

The Electromagnetic Spectrum

Non-ionizing Radiation | Ionizing Radiation

Radio | Micro Waves | Infrared | Visible Light | Ultra Violet | X-Rays | Gamma Rays | Cosmic Rays

←— Low Energy ←——→ High Energy —→

and radiation all fit on this spectrum. The spectrum is organized by frequency, with the lower frequencies to the left and the higher on the right.

Frequency is the number of occurrences of a repeating event per unit time. Frequency is measured in hertz (Hz). One Hz means the cycle repeats once a second. If a light flashes at 1 HZ then it will flash 60 times a minute.

Not only is the spectrum organized by increasing frequency, increasing frequency corresponds with decreasing wavelength.

Wavelength is a measure of the distance between repetitions of a shape feature such as peaks, valleys, or zero crossings (zero crossings are where the wave crosses the centerline of the wave, or 0 on the X axis).

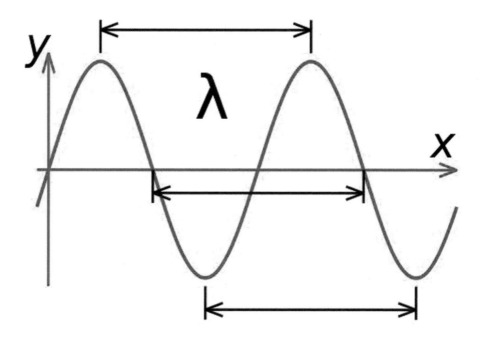

Basically the more repetitions you cram into a span of time the smaller distance you can travel. I can make ten little hops a minute easier than I can make ten standing long jumps in a minute. The distance between when my feet leave the ground to where they land is wavelength, how many I do in a span of time is frequency.

Like I said above, we tend to think of EMP coming from nuclear detonation. As a military weapon, this works best if the nuclear warhead is detonated hundreds of kilometers above Earth's surface. This is called a high-altitude electromagnetic pulse (HEMP) device. Effects of a HEMP device depend on a large number of factors, including the altitude of the detonation, energy yield, gamma ray output, interactions with Earth's magnetic field, and electromagnetic shielding of targets.

Let's talk a second about the mechanisms of injury from EMP—what the pulse does to fry your gear.

EMP works through induction—just like a transformer. When the electromagnetic energy passes by a conductor it induces the electrons inside the conductor to move—*inducing* electricity. It works just like the wall wart you use to charge your cell phone. The electricity coming from your wall at 115 volts is run into an electromagnet. This electromagnetism then induces current in a coil of wire next to the magnet—the electricity from that coil is a lower voltage and allows you to charge your cell phone.

The longer the conductor the more power is induced by a pulse. Power transmission lines, large antennas, and metal pipelines all will have induced electricity. Anything connected to those items could have a large surge of electricity in the event of an EMP.

This surge of electricity can cause problems by melting tiny wires in the electronics; large enough surges can overwhelm insulators and turn them into conductors (melting them in the process). It can also exceed a diode's breakdown voltage. This is the voltage required to reverse electrical flow in a one-way diode—basically ending its life as a diode. If this happens the circuit will not work.

Just because something does not plug into grid power does not mean it is immune to EMP—although equipment may not receive those strong induced currents, the tiny wires inside of microcircuits do not take as much current to melt so they can receive enough induced current through its internal circuits if the EMP is strong enough.

With EMP there is some confusion—not only does it come from multiple events, it comes in several different variations.

This causes certain individuals to lump things that protect against one form of EMP and believe it protects against all types of EMP.

The International Electrotechnical Commission has categorized EMP into three types.

E1

The E1 pulse is the fastest form of nuclear EMP. It is an extremely brief but very intense electromagnetic field that can quickly induce very high voltages in electrical conductors. The E1 component causes most of its damage by causing electrical breakdown voltages to be exceeded. E1 is the component that can destroy computers and communications equipment, and it changes too quickly for ordinary lightning protectors to provide effective protection against it. Lightning has a building effect where the pulse takes a few milliseconds to build and protection circuits can detect it and shut down. E1 is almost instantaneous and moves through the circuits before they can detect. Like how you slow down after the cop has you on radar . . .

The E1 component is produced when gamma radiation from the nuclear detonation knocks electrons out of the atoms in the upper atmosphere (Compton Effect).

E2

The E2 component is generated by the neutrons released by nuclear weapons. This E2 component is an "intermediate time" pulse that, by the IEC definition, lasts from about 1 microsecond to 1 second after the beginning of the electromagnetic pulse. The E2 component of the pulse has many similarities to the electromagnetic pulses produced by lightning. Because of the similarities to lightning coupled with the widespread use of lightning protection technology, the E2 pulse is generally considered to be the easiest to protect against.

However, since E2 occurs after an E1 pulse, most lightning protection equipment will probably be already damaged or destroyed.

E3

E3 is different from both E1 and E2. E3 has a very slow pulse, lasting tens to hundreds of seconds.

What happens is that after a HEMP, the earth's magnetic field is thrown out of balance by the EMP, and the molten iron core of the earth that creates our magnetic field restores itself. This causes additional induction. This is the most similar to geomagnetic storms caused by a very severe CME.

This is most likely to cause induced currents in long electrical conductors, which can then damage components such as power line transformers.

Because of the similarity between solar-induced geomagnetic storms and nuclear E3, it has become common to refer to solar-induced geomagnetic storms as "solar EMP." At ground level, however, "solar EMP" is not known to produce an E1 or E2 component.

The best way to protect against EMP is through the use of Faraday cages to shield against the pulse. Theoretically, the cages are simple.

A Faraday cage is a conductor (either solid or a mesh smaller than the height of the electromagnetic wave). This cage completely encapsulates your device. It also has an insulator inside to keep the protected items from touching the cage.

Just like a rock on the beach causing waves to flow around it, EMP hits the cage and the energy is directed around your electronics rather than through them.

Some believe the cage needs to be made out of ferrous materials, but all that is needed is that the cage is a conductor, as any conductor can make an electro-magnet.

Some also believe you need to ground your cage. Personally I disagree and feel the grounding wire will act as an antenna. However, it is possible for a conductor and an insulator to turn into a capacitor, and some believe a grounding rod will prevent this.

My biggest fear when it comes to Faraday cages is that any enemy that uses a HEMP against us will know some of us will have items that are protected, and will detonate a second EMP at some point (a week, 10 days, a month) after the initial attack to destroy our redundant systems just like an earthquake's aftershock. This coupled with the idea that Faraday cages only protect against items that are not in use and stored properly leads me to spend time in building capability in the nonelectric realm rather than spend all my resources building redundant cages stocked with redundant gear. Electronics are helpful but our civilization developed without them, and if I had to I think I can live without them (even though I am addicted to Angry Birds . . .).

EMP Protection

Now that we have covered the theory, let's work on how to put it into practical use.

You hear a lot of Internet commando ideas on Faraday cages, but you rarely see people actually test the cages they talk about. I did not build an EMP generator (mostly because of the expense, and partly because I don't want homeland security putting me on a watch list), so I had to find a reasonable alternative.

For the tests I used a cell phone and a FMRS/GMRS handle talkie. Cell phones operate in the 850/900/1800/1900 MHz ranges at about .75 to 1 watt, and FRS/GMRS is around the 463 MHz range at about 5 watts. Neither of these are within the test ranges of the 1962 HEMP tests of 1 KHz to 100

MHz but they are within the range of later tests that show EMP ranges from 200MHz—5GHz and may be as high as 30-billion watts (depending on type and distance from source). I am not trying to protect my cell phone in a post EMP area; a cell phone would be useless (except for fire building if you had steel wool).

I figure if my cage cannot shield against cell phone transmission, then it is worthless against the much higher EMP.

Personally I don't rely on any of the cages I tested, and only use them to keep a few redundant items in them to make life easier. I feel that in the event of a man-made EMP attack, the few things I can store won't balance with use versus cost, so I spend my resources on items to work around electrical dependence.

To work a Faraday cage needs to completely enclose whatever you want to protect with a conductive material. Solid metal works best, but in many cases mesh will work. (The holes in mesh will allow certain specific wavelengths through though, depending on the size of the holes). The conductive material also needs to be insulated from whatever is inside the cage; otherwise it is just an antenna.

I tried using a plastic bag inside a large Mylar bag, an ammo can, a popcorn tin, and a large garbage can. They all worked to some extent or another, even if it just reduced the range of transmission, but a large galvanized garbage can, with cardboard cut up and taped inside worked the best. Just make sure that the lid can fully seat and contact the rim of the can.

Summary

If you have completed these projects, or just some of these projects, you undoubtedly have gained confidence and skills that will serve you well during times of crisis.

You probably have also figured out that these projects are just a start, and serve a larger purpose of cultivating a "can do" attitude and the ability to think about a problem and find a solution.

This book was never about the projects themselves; it was about the journey to gain skills, and I hope you have learned as much during this journey as I have.

Keep on, and remember:

Don't Be Scared, Be Prepared.

David Nash

About the Author

David Nash is a former U.S. Marine Corps noncommissioned officer, correctional supervisor and firearms instructor for the Tennessee Department of Correction. Currently he is an emergency management planner, as well as the owner of the Shepherd School.

David has been a prepper his entire life. He started in elementary school by using every bouillon cube his mother ever brought into the house to make survival kits, creating an earthquake awareness campaign in high school, earning a degree in Emergency Management, and achieving certification as an emergency management professional.

Not only is David an avid do-it-yourselfer, he is a lifelong learner, who has completed thousands of hours of in-person training in such subjects as emergency management, response to terrorist attacks, hazardous materials, radiological response, search and rescue, and critical incident stress.

David is a state-certified hazardous material technician, law enforcement–certified firearm instructor, and crazy beekeeper.

He has written numerous articles on a wide variety of subjects, as well as the firearm manual *Understanding the Use of Handguns for Self Defense.*

You can see more of David's work on his website at http://www.tngun.com.

NOTES

NOTES